# Molecular Characterization
# Of
# Prostate Specific Antigen

**Prof.Dr. Sami A.AL-Mudhaffar**

**Ahmed Mousa Issa**

# Chapter One

## 1. Introduction

Prostate specific antigen PSA is a single chain glycoprotein with a molecular weight of 33kd[1]. It consists of 240 amino acids and 4 carbohydrate side chains[2]. It is produced by the epithelial cells lining the acini and ducts of the prostate gland[3], and under normal conditions is secreted into the lumina of the prostate ducts and can be detected in high concentrations in seminal plasma[4]. PSA function as a serine protease and is known to cause liquefaction of seminal coagulum[5]. The gene in coding PSA is located on the long arm of chromosome 19 in human[6]. PSA was originally identified in seminal plasma in 1971[7]. Purified in 1972[8], and isolated from human prostate tissue in 1979 and named prostate specific antigen[9]. A serologic test followed in 1980[10]. It is currently measured with commercial immunoassays that use monoclonal antibodies to identify epitopes on the PSA molecule.

PSA is prostate specific, not prostate cancer specific as such, PSA level is can be elevated by any prostatic disease: Prostatitis, BPH, prostate cancer, and prostate manipulation[11]. The levels of PSA are dependent on the volume of cancer present, the volume of BPH in the prostate, and the histologic differentiation. These factors have an important implications in using PSA in staging and diagnosis[12].

In most reports, further diagnostic is advised if the serum PSA value exceeds 4ng.ml$^{-1}$[13]. In spite of the development of PSA, it is difficult to differentially diagnose prostate carcinoma and BPH in patients with intermediate serum PSA level 4-10ng.ml$^{-1}$[11].

Several modifications to the PSA test have been proposed to improve its specificity: PSA density[14], PSA velosity[15], the use of age specific PSA reference ranges[16], and free PSA to total PSA ratio[17] have been evaluated.

The pathophysiology of the delivery of PSA from prostate tissue in to circulation is not yet understood, but because PSA is normally secreted into the ejaculation, its appearance in serum indicate leakage[18]. The accessibility of PSA to circulation from each tumor is the factor that control the relationship between PSA concentration and tumor grade[19]. The high concentration of PSA might favor the growth of cells especially the formation of metastases[20]. Like other protease, PSA may facilitate prostate cancer cell invasion and metastasis[21]. Further more, a weak stimulation of growth of prostate stroma cells and prostate epithelial cells was identified for PSA, despite the fact that the receptor for this molecule has not yet been discovered[22].

Serum PSA levels after radical prostatectomy are an important indicator of persistent carcinoma. For patients undergoing radical prostatectomy serum PSA levels exceeding $0.5ng.ml^{-1}$ for 2-3 months post prostatectomy indicate the presence of residual microscopic disease, leading ultimately to recurrence[23]. Many publications have confirmed that PSA is widely expressed, at lower concentrations than in prostate in many tissues, especially in female breast[24]. PSA has been detected in all pathological breast secretions, tissue extracts, and fluids (milk, breast cyst fluid, nipple aspirate fluids); but these new finding do not limit the value of PSA in prostate cancer diagnosis but may expands its application to breast cancer[24].

PSA is present in human blood as a complex mixture of several species. The main immunologically detectable form is a covalent complex of PSA with the serine protease inhibitor $\alpha_1$- anti chymotrypsin[25]. Complex of PSA with $\alpha_2$-macroglobulin is also present, but it has not been detected by clinically used immunological tests and, therefore, does not contribute to the PSA values measured by these tests[26]. Free PSA is also present accounting for 5-30% of total PSA in serum. This PSA form is enzymatically inactive and can not form complexes with protease inhibitors[27]. The ratio of free to total PSA and also the ratio of free PSA to PSA-ACT complex is being used for better differentiation between prostate cancer and BPH than total PSA alone[28].

Prostate cancer patients have a high proportion of PSA-ACT and a low proportion of free PSA, compared with normal population and with BPH patients[29]. The PSA-ACT complex is readily detected in serum but not in prostatic fluid or in seminal plasma[30]. The ratio of free to total PSA is constant with aging, and therefore, should be available parameter for measurement regardless of patients age[31]. The free PSA seems to be stable upon frozen, storage and show a negligible effect when interfering substances are added to serum[32].

## 2. The Prostate:

The prostate is a complex organ composed of branching tubuloalveolar glands that eventually enter the prostatic urethra. They are arranged in lobules and surrounded by stroma. Its located in the plevis and is surrounded by the rectum posteriorly, the bladder superiorily, dorsal sphincter interiorly[33]. The gland is made up of five zones. The transition zone that surrounds the prostatic urethra occupies 5% of the glandular tissue, yet 20% of cancers develop in this region. Central zone that surrounds the prostatic ejaculatory ducts occupies 15-20% of the gland, yet only 5-10% of prostate cancer occurs here. The peripheral zone that surrounds the central zone, consists of 70% of prostate gland and 70% of cancers occur in this location[34].

Periurethral glands lie adjacent to the urethra and are surrounded by the proximal sphincter, carcinomas do not arise from these glands which represent the fourth zone. Finally the fibromusclar stroma, primarily muscle, occupies the anterior surface of the prostate[34].

## 3. Biological Properties of Prostate Gland:

Human prostate gland consists of epithelial cells and stromal cells. Epithelial cells involves three types of cells: secretory glandular cells, nonsecretory basal cells, and neuroendocrine cells[35].

Secretory glandular cells contain androgen receptors on their surfaces, are androgen dependent for growth, synthesise and secretion of PSA and PAP, both of which are mixed with prostatic fluids of ejaculation[35].

The nonsecretory basal cell lack androgen receptors and are thought to be stem cells for secretory epithelial cells[36]. The stroma of the prostate is composed of smooth muscle cells, fibroblasts, lymphocyte, and neuromuscular tissue cells. Evidence suggested that epithelial-stromal interactions play an important role in normal prostatic growth[37].

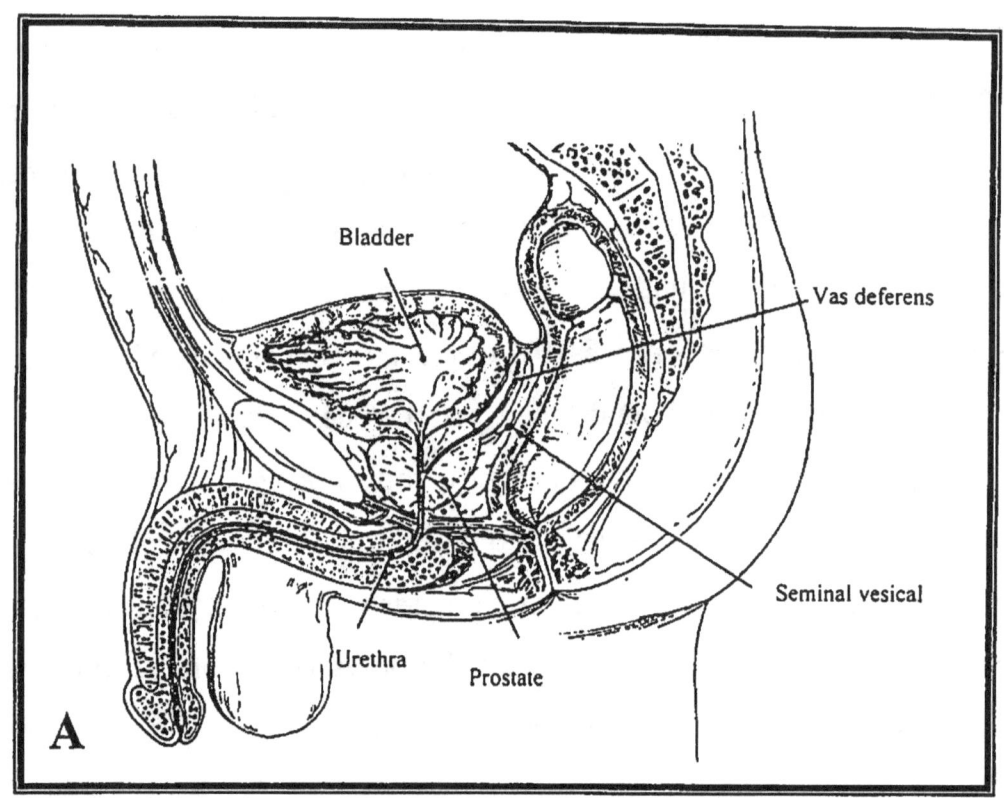

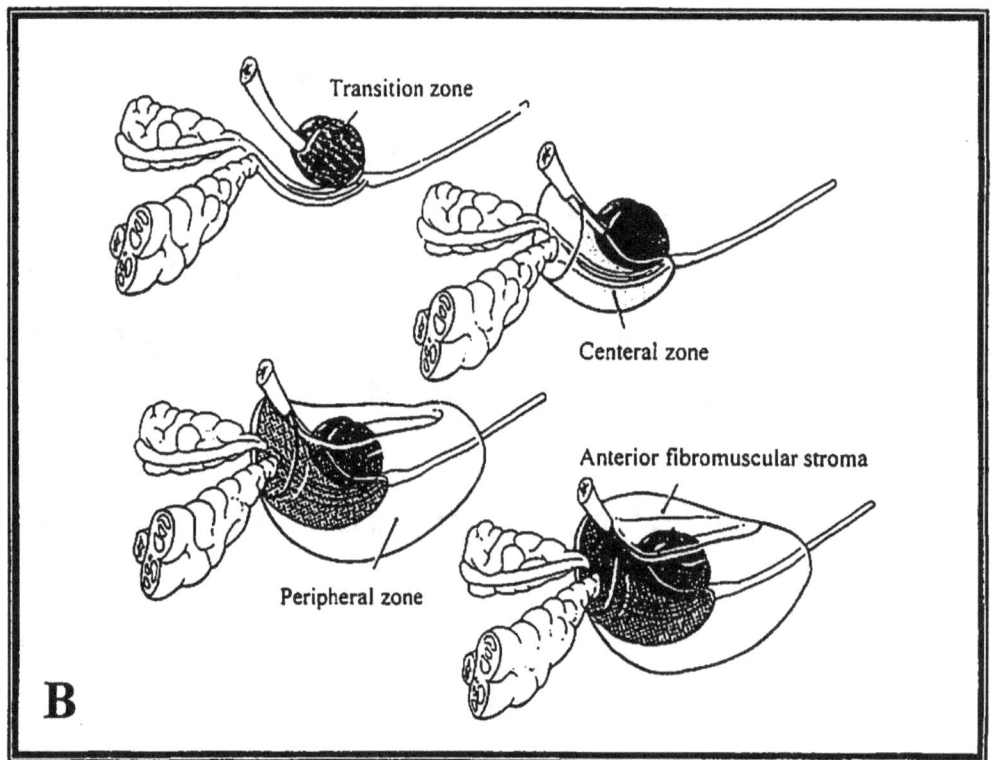

*Figure (1-1): A- Human prostate location.*

*B- Zonal anatomy of prostate gland[34].*

## 4. Prostate Cancer:

Carcinogenesis of prostate is a multistep accumulation of genetic lesions that may result in uncontrolled cellular proliferation, a decrease in cell death or apoptosis, invasion, metastatic spread and blockade of prostatic cell differentiation[38]. In the prostate, the expression of the malignant phenotype represents the balance of the expression of oncogene driven malignant conversion and expression of tumor supressor genes that inhibit this process[39]. The two well- known risk factors for developing prostate cancer are increased aging and the presence of gonadal androgenic hormone[40]. The androgen has been shown to regulate the expression of many prostatic growth factors and androgen ablation is the most common first –line treatment for prostate cancer patients[41].

Other factors recently studied include hereditary and familial factors (genetic predisposibilty)[42], African- American descent[43], high fat diet[44], smoking and alcohol intake[45], sexual relationships, prior vasectomy[36], and vitamin D deficiency[46] all are still controversial.

## 5. Incidence:

Prostate cancer is the most common cancer and cause of death in men older than age 55 years[47].

It is rare before the age of 40 years, and incidence increases there after with advancing age. More than 60% of the cases occur in man older than 70 years. Moreover, there is now a good evidence that only about 10% of all cases identified at autopsy are detected during lifetime[48].

In 2000 about 180,000 new cases were diagnosed and nearly 31,900 patients had died of prostate cancer in USA [49]. In Iraq table (1-1) shows the numbers of diagnosed cases with prostate cancer within the period 1987-1997[50].

*Table (1-1): Number of Diagnosed Cases of Prostate Cancer in Iraq During (1987-1997) Interval*

| Year | Number of diagnosed cases | Year | Number of diagnosed cases |
|------|---------------------------|------|---------------------------|
| 1987 | 99 | 1993 | 160 |
| 1988 | 132 | 1994 | 137 |
| 1989 | 130 | 1995 | 135 |
| 1990 | 117 | 1996 | 152 |
| 1991 | 126 | 1997 | 150 |
| 1992 | 146 | | |

In Asian countries the proportion of patients with prostate carcinoma is much smaller than in western countries. There are wide geographical and racial differences in the incidence of prostatic cancer, ranging from 1 case per 100,000 population in Asia to 100 per 100,000 among black population in the United State[48].

# 6.Pathological Classification of Prostate Neoplasm:

prostatic neoplasm can be classified to epithelial and nonepithelial neoplasm over 99% of cancers that develop in the prostate are adenocarcinomas derived from epithelial cells[51]. Other type of epithelial neoplasms are small cell tumors and transitional cell carcinoma[52]. Non epithelial neoplasm is represent by malignant mesenchymal tumors which makeup less than 0.3% of prostatic neoplasm and lymphoma. There is also a third type of prostatic neoplasm, the carcinosarcoma which defined as the coexistence of histologically differentiated carcinoma plus malignant of mesenchymal elements[53].

# 7.Stages and Grades of Prostate Cancer:

Table (1-2) shows the American urological system for prostate cancer staging.

*Table (1-2): American Staging System of Prostate Cancer[54]*

| American urological system (A –D) | |
|---|---|
| Stage A | incidental finding |
| Stage B | confined to prostate |
| Stage C | localized to periprostatic area |
| Stage D | metastatic disease |

The most important aspect in prostate cancer staging is the distinction between stage B and stage C. This distinction represents the border line between treatment and surgery choice. Surgery is not recommended for patients with clinical stage C disease. The DRE is insufficient and inaccurate in this field. TRUS also lacks sensitivity and specificity while CT was not better[55]. MRI applied either trans abdominally or transrectally and offers a modest improvement for staging[56].

Gleason system is the most widely utilized grading system to determine the biologic potential of prostate tumors. The high score of this system is 10 and its represent the undifferentiated tumors with virtually complete loss of the glandular architecture while the low score 2 reflects the most differentiated tumor with discrete glandular formation[57].

## 8. Signs and Symptoms of Prostate Cancer:

The peripheral zone cancer does not produce symptoms in early stages. Those that arise in the transition zone may produce hesitancy, a decrease in the force of the urinary stream and intermittency. The later obstruction may results in bladder instability and this in turn can produce symptoms of urinary frequency, nocturia and urgency incontinence. Progression to the seminal vesicle can result in hematospermia or a decrease in the volume of the ejaculate. Invasive of the neurovascular bundles can produce impotence[58].

## 9. Diagnosis of Prostate Cancer:

The diagnosis of prostate cancer is based on symptoms, and abnormal DRE or elevated serum PSA levels, and established by TRUS-guided transrectal needle biopsy (TRNB) using a biopsy gun[59]. CT is not recommended to detect localized lesion of prostate while, MRI is useful in imaging the periprostatic fat, periprostatic venous plexus, perivesiclar tissue, lumph nodes and bone marrow and are most useful in demonstrating the internal architecture of prostate and seminal vesicle[60].

## 10. Treatment of Prostate Cancer:

The methods of treatment of prostate cancer involve the following:

◆ Surgery:

Tumors that confined to prostate stage A and B are generally managed by radical surgery. In the early stages the radical prostatectomy may be curative. The outcome with radical prostatectomy alone for stage C tumors are very poor[61].

◆ Radiation:

Locally advanced clinical stage C and stage D tumors are generally treated by external beam radiation alone or in combination with androgen ablation. Delivery of tumoricidal dose level by a penetrating megavoltage beams directed to the prostate tumors without excessive damage to the skin and normal tissues surrounding the prostate is represent the basic tenet of radiotherapy of prostate cancer[62].

## ◆ Hormonal Treatment:

The hormonal treatment of prostate cancer may involve the following:

### ▪ Bilateral Orchiectomy:

The basic treatment for advanced prostate cancer is the bilateral orchiectomy. Its surgery to remove the testicle, which are the main source of male hormones[63].

### ▪ Estrogens:

Exogenous estrogens inhibit lutenizing hormone- releasing hormone (LHRH) production from the hypothalamus, which regulates lutenizing hormone and follicle- stimulating hormone (FSH) release from pituitary. LH and FSH acts to increase spermatogenesis and androgen production[64]. Such as goserelin.

### ▪ Progestational Agents:

The progestational agent supress LH release from pituitary gland and inhibit intracellular binding of dihydrotestosterone (DHT) to the androgen receptor[65].

### ▪ Gonadotropin- Releasing Hormone Analogues:

These compounds are analogues of LHRH. They initially produce arise in LH and FSH. This is followed by a down regulation of receptors in the pituitary, which results in a chemical castration. Such as buserelin[66].

### ▪ Adrenal Enzyme Synthesis Inhibitors.

Agents that inhibit adrenal androgen synthesis enzymes are usually administered as second line therapy, in untreated patients the administration of these inhibitors may results in chemical castration in less than 24 hours. Such as ketocanazole and aminoglutethimide[67].

- **Anti androgens:**

   Anti androgens compete with androgens for sites on the androgens receptor. Such as flutamide and bicalutamide[68].

- **Combined Androgen Blockade (CAB):**

   Although castration, (medical or surgical), causes a reduction of about 90% in serum testosterone concentration, the androgen biosynthesis in the adrenal, which contributes 8-10% of the total amount of androgens is not affected. This illustrates the extra benefit of CAB by the addition of anti androgens to castration (medical or surgical) to create a completely free milieu[69].

# 11. Tumor Markers of Prostate Cancer:

Tumor markers are substances that reflect genesis, growth and response to therapy of malignant tumors and that either produced by the tumor cells or by cells of the host stimulated by tumor disease[70]. The optimal tumor marker for prostate would be effective for early detection, staging, and monitoring patients after definitive treatment. The tumor marker would have sensitivity, specificity, and positive predictive value for distinguishing men with prostate cancer. It would detect biologically significant disease, correlate with clinical and pathologic staging, predict prognosis and provide an indication of disease activity following treatment. From a practical standpoint it should also be reproducible, inexpensive, easy to administer accessible, and tolerable to patients[71].

There are two important tumor markers in prostate cancer. The prostate specific antigen (PSA) which fulfills many of the previous requirements[9] and prostatic acid phosphatase the enzyme that was used extensively prior to the discovery of prostate specific antigen for the diagnosis, staging and monitoring of patients with prostate cancer[72]. Table (1-3) shows the position of these tumor markers among other most used tumor markers.

*Table (1-3): Some Relevant Tumor Markers for Drivers Tumors [38].*

| Enzymes | Hormones | Proteins | Antigens |
|---|---|---|---|
| LDH- Iso enzymes | Gastrin | B2- Microglobulin | CEA |
| | Insulin | Calcitonin | AFP |
| CK- Iso enzymes | Glucagon | Thyroglobulin | CA 19-9 |
| Pancreas Elastase | VIP | HCG | CA 50 |
| Phosphohexose- Isomerase | Serotonine | | CA 195 |
| Prostate specific antigen | Pancreatic poly peptide | | CA 125 |
| Neuron- specific Enolase | Neurotensin | | CA 15-3 |
| Thymidin- Kinase | Somatostatin | | PSA |
| Prostatic acid phosphatase | Adrenaline | | |
| Placental Alkaline phasphatase | Cortisol | | |

## 12.Prostate Specific Antigen (PSA):

Prostate specific antigen is a 33 Kd glycoprotein that belongs to the kallikrein serine protease family. PSA molecular weight of peptide moity is 26.079 kd[1]. The four carbohydrate side chain linkage at aminoacids 45 (aspargine), 69 (serine), 70 (alanine) and 71 serine. The N- terminal aminoacid is isoleucine while the C- terminal residue is proline[73]. It's a single chain expressed predominantly by the secretory epithelial cell lining the acini and ducts of the human prostate. After PSA is secreted to the lumen of the prostate gland, it becomes a constituent of seminal fluid[3]. It contains about 240 amino acid residues, the molecular features 7-10% carbohydrate contents, isoelectric point at PH 6.8-7.5, sedimentation coefficient 3.1 S[2]. There are at least five PSA isoforms based on different isoelectric point have been described. These isoenzymes may differ in their carbohydrate position ranging from non-glycosylated to fully glycosylated structure[74].

## 13.Physiological Aspect of Prostate Specific Antigen:

PSA is one of the major proteins of seminal plasma the essential function of PSA is to liquefy the sperm entrapping seminal coagulum after ejaculation[4]. The seminal substrates of PSA, a serine protease with chymotrypsin- like specificity, are the major structural constituents of gel- like coagulum seminogelin I, seminogelin II, and fibronectin. These proteins are degraded to small peptides and soluble fragments by PSA, thereby increasing spermatozoa motility[5]. PSA has been shown to cleave other biological substrates, including insulin- like growth factor indicating the potential role of PSA in the regulation of various biological functions[75].

The gene that encodes for PSA is located on the long arm of chromosome 19[6]. Its synthesized as a 261 amino acid preproform from which the 17- amino acid single peptide is cleaved in the secretion process then, the remaining zymogen form of PSA is activated to an active serine protease enzyme by cleavage of the 7 aminoacid of propeptide[76]. In prostatic epithelial cells the expression of PSA gene is under complex control and the steady- state level of PSA, m RNA is increased by androgens and decreased by epidermal growth factor and activation of protein kinase C. These changes suggest the existence of many regulatory elements in control the expression of PSA gene[77]. Only trace amounts of PSA leak into the blood of healthy males, normally its concentration found to be lower than 2.5 ng. ml$^{-1}$ but, vary according to human age[78].

In 1990, the discovery was made that PSA exists in different forms when found in the systemic circulation. Probably the most promising development in enhancing the performance of PSA testing involves measuring the different molecular forms of PSA proteins in serum[25]. It was determined that PSA in serum has a tendency to form irreversibly and covalently complexes with $\alpha_1$-anti chymotrypsin (ACT) an endogenous serine protease inhibitor and this form is enzymatically inactive. Smaller quantities of PSA are also complexed to $\alpha 2$-macroglobulin (AMG) in particular[26]. PSA can however remain in a free unbound state. Furthermore, five distinct immunoreactive epitopes have been identified on the free uncomplexed PSA molecule available for immunoreactive detection of serum level[27]. Figure (1-2) shows these three forms and how some of the epitopes are masked when complex forms. The PSA- ACT complex for example, covers three of the epitopes of PSA leaving two available to react with antibodies, thus PSA- ACT and free PSA are two molecular forms that may be monitored using immunological methods such as immunoassays.

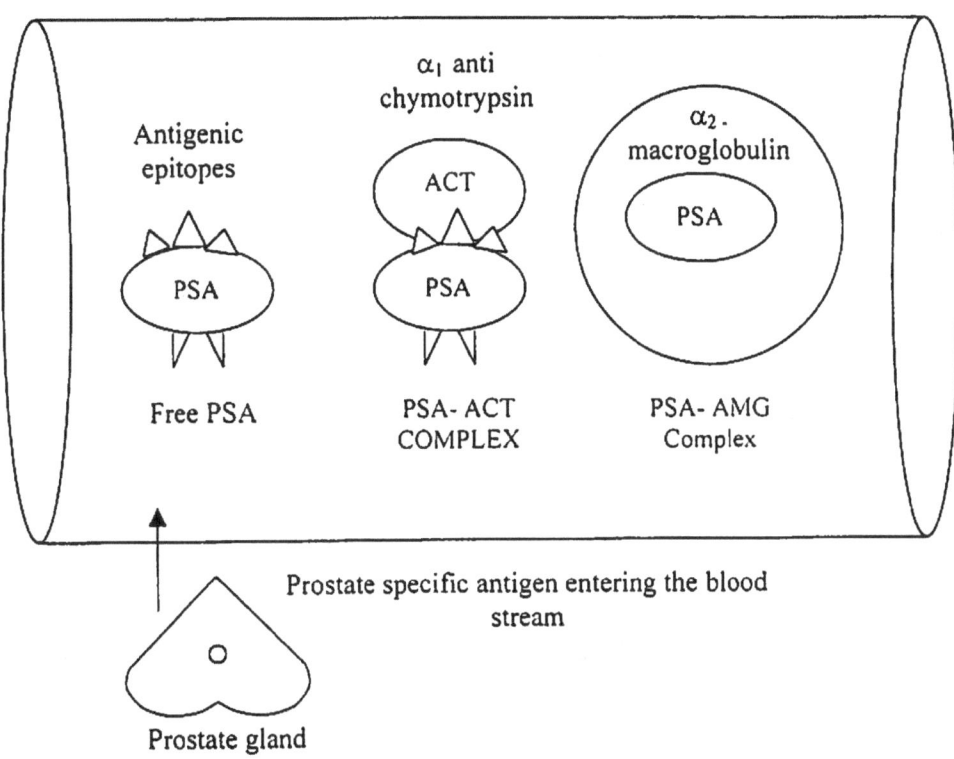

*Figure (1-2): Illustration of the three molecular forms of PSA while in the systemic circulation[57].*

The PSA- AMG complex covers all of the antigenic regions and is therefore not detected by conventional immunoassays[80]. PSA in serum should be considered a biologically active factor, however its enzymatic activity in serum may exhibit a certain growth- factor like effect. The enzyme activity of PSA in blood possesses mitogenic activity[81], may be involved in growth regulation[82] and in higher concentration might favor the growth of cells especially the formation of metastases[20]. Other investigators have reported that PSA can release kinin- like substance that simulate smooth muscle contraction by digesting a glycoproteins present in seménal vesicle fluid[83]. Webber *et al*[21] put forward the idea that like other proteases, PSA may facilitate prostate cancer cell invasion and metastasis. Furthermore, a weak stimulation of growth of prostate stroma cells and prostate epithelial cells was identified for PSA, despite the fact that the receptor for this molecule has not yet been discovered[22].

## 14. Pathological Aspect of Prostate Specific Antigen:

The pathophysiology of the delivery of PSA from prostate tissue into circulation is not yet understood, but because PSA is normally secreted into the ejaculation, its appearance in serum indicate leakage[18]. High concentration of PSA can be detected in the blood of patients with prostate cancer and benign prostatic hyperplasia and various other urological problems[84]. Although PSA considered effective tumor marker and for practical purposes organ specific, it is not cancer specific. There is a considerable overlap in PSA concentration in men with prostate cancer and men with benign prostatic disease, particularly in the range of 4-10 ng.ml$^{-1}$. This range has thus been termed the diagnostic gray zone[11]. Serum level of PSA is normally below 4.0 ng.ml$^{-1}$ however any process disrupts the normal architecture of the prostate gland allows diffusion of PSA in to stroma and microvasculature. Elevated serum PSA levels are seen in a variety of prostatic diseases with elevation of greatest clinical importance in prostate adenocarcinoma[85].

Cancer produces less PSA per cell than benign epithelial but greater number of malignant cells and stromal disrubtion associated with cancer account for the elevated serum PSA level[86]. There is a suggestion that PSA enters the circulation from prostatic epithelial cells after the basement membrane breakdown, an early event in prostatic cancer. The accessibility of PSA to circulation from each tumor is the factor that control the relationship between PSA concentration and tumor grade[19]. The tumors that causing elevated serum PSA are more likely to have large cancer volume, higher pathological grade (poorly differentiated) and more advanced pathological stage than tumors with normal serum PSA levels[87]. PSA levels correlate positivity with clinical stage, histological grade and presence of capsular perforation and seminal vesicle invasion. Its also predict the presence of lymphnode metastases, bone metastases and survival after androgen deprivation therapy[86]. Serum PSA levels after radical prostatectomy are an important indicator of persistent carcinoma. For patients undergoing radical prostatectomy serum PSA levels exceeding 0.5 ng.ml$^{-1}$ for 2 to 3 months postprostatectomy indicate the presence of residual microscopic disease, leading ultimately to recurrence[23]. Its also reported that serial PSA determinations were useful to assess the disease status of patient treated with radiotherapy for prostate cancer[88]. The different occurrence of free and combined PSA forms in the serum of prostate cancer and BPH patients and the use of free PSA total PSA ratio is a promising discriminatory tool between both groups of patients. It has been postulated that PSA is more extensively complexes in prostate cancer than in non diseased prostate or BPH[89]. Consequently, the lower free PSA/ total PSA ratio in serum of prostate cancer patients compared with BPH has been assumed to reflect cellular peculiarility after PSA is released into the blood stream[90]. However, many publications have confirmed that PSA is widely expressed, at lower concentrations than in prostate, in many tissues, especially in female breast[24]. PSA has been detected in all pathological breast secretions, tissue extracts, and fluids (milk, breast cyst fluid, nipple aspirate fluid). These new findings do not limit the value of PSA in prostate cancer diagnosis but may expand its applications to breast cancer[91].

## 15.Prostate Specific Antigen Specificity and Sensitivity:

Measuring serum PSA levels, in addition to preforming digital rectal examination (DRE), can effectively detect prostate cancer at curable stage in a majority of men[92]. Despite the impressive yield of a serum PSA greater than 4.0 ng.ml$^{-1}$ as an indication for further work up, many patients exceeding this cut off value and have a negative biopsy[13]. The lack of specificity evidenced by fact that two out of three men with

PSA greater than 4.0 ng.ml$^{-1}$ do not have carcinoma on initial biopsy[93]. A considerable efforts have directed to improve the performance of this most important of all tumor markers.

The diagnostic performance of clinical testing is usually evaluated in terms of sensitivity, specificity, positive predictive value (PPV) and negative predictive value (NPV)[94]. In practical terms, the sensitivity is the measure of test ability to find disease in patients that actually have it.

$$\text{Sensitivity} = \frac{\text{no. of true positive}}{\text{no. of true positive} + \text{no. of false negative}}$$

The specificity of a test reflects the likelihood that the disease is absent if the test is negative[95].

$$\text{Specificity} = \frac{\text{no. of true negative}}{\text{no. of true negative} + \text{no. of false positive}}$$

The sensitivity and specificity of PSA tests are inversely proportional[96]. The sensitivity and specificity altered with the variation of serum PSA cut – off value[97]. If a lower PSA cut – off values were used, a large number of cancers would be detected (increase sensitivity) but more men would be required to undergo prostate biopsy due to falsely elevated PSA value (reduce specificity). Like wise, as efforts are directed at increasing the specificity of PSA, a resultant decrease in the sensitivity would be expected. The most efficient cut– off point for a given test would provide the greatest sensitivity and specificity[98]. There are many methods to improve the performance of PSA testing for the diagnosis of prostate cancer.

## 15.1. Prostrate Specific Antigen Density:

The specificity of serum PSA testing could be enhanced by measuring the prostate specific antigen density (PSAD), which was describe as the result of serum PSA divided by the volume of prostate gland, the units for PSAD would by ng.ml$^{-1}$.ml$^{-1}$[14]. In addition, serum PSA levels shows a significant correlation with tumor volume and appears to be correlated well with cancer volume. PSA cancer density increased reliability and predictive value of pathological stage[99]. MRI and later TRUS was used to measure prostate volume. The PSAD was an important tool in differentiation between patients who had cancer and who had BPH[100]. The investigators recommend that if the DRE was normal and the serum PSA level was between 4.0 and 10.0 ng.ml$^{-1}$ the patient should undergo TRUS to determine the volume of the prostate. If there is any elevation in PSAD a systematic prostate biopsy should be performed[101]. Although, the measurement of the size of prostate gland using transrectal ultrasound involves costly procedure, the PSAD value may provide a useful information for the patient that initially presents with elevated serum PSA or abnormal digital rectal examination[97].

## 15.2. Prostate Specific Antigen Velocity:

Prostate specific antigen velocity (PSAV) is the rate of change in serum PSA concentration over time[15]. The serial PSA measurements used to evaluate the rate of change would provide insight into detecting cancer[102]. PSAV, in theory, would be potentially important tool for monitoring the status of prostate in patients who truly do not have cancer, as well as those who are harboring incidental tumors that may not have become clinically manifest[103]. Patients with BPH had a linear increase in PSA velocity, whereas patients with cancer initially had linear increase in PSA with subsequent exponential rise by using this information as an approach to enhance detection, a significant improvement in the specificity and sensitivity will be possible[104].

## 15.3. Age Specific Prostate Specific Antigen Reference Range:

Age specific reference ranges make use of the observation that prostate specific antigen levels increase with age[16]. The change in the diagnostic performance associated with using age – specific PSA cut- off values was appreciated[105]. For men younger than 60 years old with a negative DRE, a lower cut- off value translates to a large number of cancers being detected (greater sensitivity) but with an increase in the number of biopsy required (reduce specificity) as compared with utilizing well established cut- off value 4 ng.ml$^{-1}$. Moreover applying age specific cut- off values for men older than 60 years with negative DRE, would produce the opposite effect[106]. The advantage of age specific reference ranges is that they increase sensitivity PSA in younger men and increase the specificity of PSA in older men[107].

## 15.4. Percentage Free- To- Total Prostate Specific Antigen:

Many studies demonstrate that measuring the free to total PSA ratio had the potential to enhance the performance of PSA testing [17,28]. The ratio between free to total PSA is constant with aging and therefore should be a valuable parameter for measurement regardless of patients age[31]. Furthermore, the free PSA seems to be stable upon frozen storage and show negligible effect when interfering substances are added to serum[32].

The most appropriate ratio to determine clinically whether a biopsy should be performed has yet to be established but some reports have utilized ranges between 0.14 and 0.25[108-110] as a cut- off values. Its possible to say that using free- to- total ratio will ensure a high sensitivity while enhances the specificity such that nearly 30% of unnecessary biopsy will prevented[111].

# 16.Clinical Utility of Prostate Specific Antigen:

## 16.1. Detection:

PSA concentration if compared with DRE as a tool for prostate cancer detection, shows a higher cancer detection rate[112]. However in most reports, if PSA concentration exceeds 4 ng.ml$^{-1}$ a further diagnostic testing is advised such as DRE and TRUS[113,114]. The developments in PSA regarding its use as a diagnostic marker have led to diagnostic algorithms to aid clinical in providing the most thorough, yet cost-effective, evaluation in prostate gland. Figure (1-3) shows the diagnostic algorithm[115].

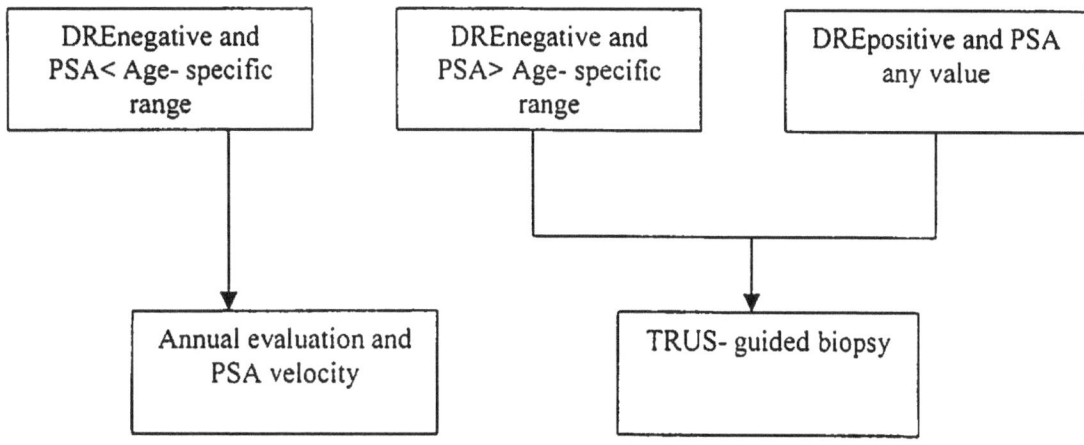

*Figure (1-3): Algorithm for the use of age- specific PSA for the detection of clinically significant prostate cancers at early, curable stage.*[115]

## 16.2. Staging:

A critical issue in staging is whether a tumor is organ confined. In general the overlap between a given PSA concentration and tumor stage preclude the reliable prediction of pathologic for the individual patient using PSA alone[116]. However, by combining the PSA concentration with the clinical findings on DRE and histologic grade on biopsy, anomograms developed to construct probability plots, to predict the probability of capsular penetration, seminal vesicle involvement and nodal involvement[117].

## 16.3. Monitoring:

The greatest clinical values of PSA appear in follow up and monitoring treatment response in patients with proven prostate cancer[118]. After radical prostatectomy, PSA concentration fall to undetectable levels according to its serum half- life value which was reported by many investigation to be 4.2 days[119]. PSA levels should have reached baseline concentrations three weeks after prostatectomy[120]. Persisting PSA levels indicate the presence of residual cancer tissue and further therapy should be considered. More over PSA levels reflect response to radiation and hormonal therapy[121].

# The aim of the work

The aim of this thesis may be summarized by the following points:-

- Determination of PSA levels in tissue and sera of Iraqi patients with prostate cancer by IRMA, and then compared with the results of age-matched control group and patients with BPH.

- Determination of PSA levels in sera of patients with prostate cancer and BPH, and then compared with the normal levels.

- Exploration the clinical importance of PSA in evaluating outcome after surgery of prostate cancer.

- Development of a method for determination PSA levels in prostate cancer tissue by studying the $^{125}$I-anti total PSA Antibody binding with PSA.

- Molecular characterization of the binding of $^{125}$I-anti total PSA antibody with PSA in prostate cancer tissue such as binding capacity and the effect of some other factors like temperature, time, pH, salt, and reactants concentration.

- Determination of kinetic and thermodynamic parameters of the binding reaction between PSA of prostate cancer tissue and $^{125}$I-anti total PSA antibody.

- Isolation of the free PSA from sera of patients with prostate cancer then, determination of the free PSA/ total PSA ratio in different stages of prostate cancer.

- Determination of kinetic and thermodynamic parameters of free PSA in sera of patients with prostate cancer and compare them with those of PSA in tissue.

- Determination of zinc levels in sera and tissue of prostate cancer using the electro thermal atomic absorption spectrophotometric method, to evaluate the relationship between zinc levels and free PSA/ total PSA ratio.

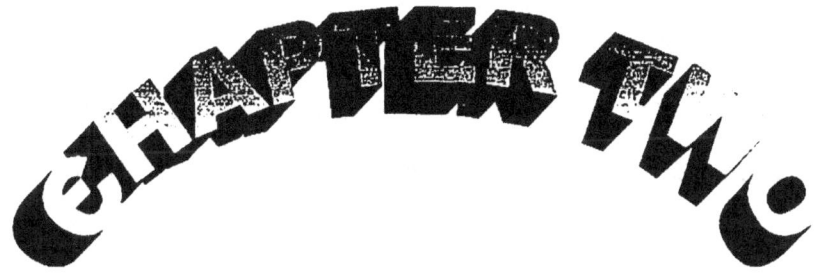

# DEVELOPMENT OF A METHOD
# FOR DETERMINATION OF
# PROSTATE SPECIFIC ANTIGEN
# IN
# PROSTATE TUMOR
# AND ITS BINDING
# KINETICS AND THERMODYNAMICS

# 1.Introduction:

RIA and IRMA which use radioactive isotopes and other methods, which use enzymes and fluorescent label are commercially available for PSA level determination. The determination of total PSA by immunoreactive methods involves the determination of free-PSA and PSA that combined $\alpha_1$- antichymotrypsin but not PSA that included in $\alpha_2$-macroglobulin which is non- immunoreactive by these methods[122].

Commercially available assays fall in two broad categories based on their relative ability to detect those two immunologically active forms of PSA: equimolar assays and nonequimolar assays[123]. Equimolar assays measures both Free–PSA and PSA combined $\alpha_1$-antichymotrypsin (PSA-ACT) equally, and results obtained by these assays are largely independent on the relative amounts of free-PSA and PSA-ACT in the test media, In contrast skewed-response assays or non-equimolar assays preferentially recognize the free from of PSA, thus measuring apparently higher total-PSA concentrations when the proportion of free-PSA increase[124]. Some of the well known assays for total PSA determination are mentioned.

Many earliest studies of PSA used the ProceCheck assay as a traditional RIA approach. Rabbit polyclonal antibodies against PSA are used to bind radioactivity labeled PSA and the PSA in the patient sample. After overnight incubation, a second goat anti rabbit antibody precipitates the primary antibody-PSA complex. The detection limit of this assay is reported to be $0.2$ng. ml$^{-1}$[125].

While the Tandem-R or tandem-E assay is a solid phase two site immunometric assay IRMA that uses two Monoclonal antibodies directed against different epitopes on the PSA molecule. Tandem-Ruses radio active label whereas Tandem-E uses alkaline phosphates label. PSA's detection limit is $0.1ng.ml^{-1}$ and a high dose (Hook) effect is observed at approximately $5000ng.ml^{-1(126)}$.

In IMX assay the automated IMX analyzer uses microparticles coated monoclonal antibodies against PSA on the solid phase to capture PSA. Alkaline phosphates linked polyclonal (goat) antibodies bound to other sites to form a sandwich- like complex. The particles bound reactants separated from other media constituents by filtration. The substrate 4-methylum belliferyl phosphate is converted to the florescent product 4-methylum bellifron. The detection limit is $0.1ng.ml^{-1}$. No high does hook effect was seen at $50000ng.ml^{-1(127)}$. Accordingly, this chapter deals with a developed method from IRMA to produce a mean to determine the kinetic and thermodynamic parameters of the reaction between serum or tissue PSA and its antibody.

## 2. Material and Methods.

### 2.1. Chemicals:

All laboratory chemicals and reagents were of analar grade

| | | |
|---|---|---|
| Tris(hydroxmethyl) amino methane | From | Fluka-Switzerland |
| Dithiothreitol | From | BDH-UK |
| EDTA | From | Fluka-Switzerland |
| Poly ethylene glycol-10000 | From | BDH-UK |
| Bovine serum albumin (BSA) | From | Sigma-USA |

| Glycerol | From | BDH-UK |
|---|---|---|
| NaCl | From | BDH-UK |
| KCl | From | BDH-UK |
| NaI | From | BDH-UK |
| NaBr | From | BDH-UK |
| NaF | From | BDH-UK |
| $MgCl_2$ | From | Fluka-Switzerland |
| $CaCl_2$ | From | Fluka-Switzerland |
| $ZnCl_2$ | From | Fluka-Switzerland |
| $CuSO_4. 5H_2O$ | From | Fluka-Switzerland |
| Na-K-tartarate | From | Fluka-Switzerland |
| HCl | From | BDH-UK |
| $Na_2CO_3$ | From | BDH-UK |
| NaOH | From | BDH-UK |
| Folin Ciocalteau reagent | From | BDH-UK |

Total PSA kit purchased from Immunotech-Beckman Coulter company-Czech Republic.

## 2.2. Apparatus

The apparatus used during this study were:

- Cold room (Combicold rack II)
- LKB gamma counter type 1270-rack gamma II.
- Pye. unicam pH meter.
- Cooling centrifuge. Type Hettich.
- Memmert incubator
- Memmert water bath
- Orbital shaker (envrion-shaker)
- Vortex (Hook)
- Heater and magnetic stirrer (scientific)

## 2.3. Patients:

Three groups of patients were included in this study. First group was involved 36 patients of different stages of prostate cancer. The second group was contained 52 patients with BPH, while the third group was included 41 individual matched with the two groups and considered as control. All these patients were admitted for treatment to Saddam Medical City, Al-Shaheed Adnan hospital, and Saddam general hospital in Al-Najaf city. They were clinically diagnosed by physicians and histologically proven by laboratory reports and were not taken any type of therapy. Patients suffered from any diseases that may interfere with our study were excluded.

## 2.4. Blood Sampling:

Venous blood samples about 5ml were collected from these patients and healthy volunteers in tubes containing no additive. The blood samples were collected before surgery (except those for postoperative monitoring) or any treatment to avoid any effect on the obtained results. A 5ml of venous blood were weekly collected from three post operative patients after surgery. After allowing the blood to clot at room temperature for about 15min, blood samples were centrifuged at 1600xg for 15min. The samples were aliquoted and frozen at $-20\ ^0C$ so as to avoid freezing and thawing for many times.

## 2.5. Collection of Specimens and Preparation of Tissue Homogentes :

The tumor tissues were surgically removed from tumor patients. Specimen were cut of and stored immediately at $-20^0$C. prior to the study, the frozen tissue was pulverized on ice path at 4C in TED buffer pH 7.4 with 1:5 weight/volume ratio. (TED buffer contains 0.01M tris (hydroxymethel) aminomethan, 0.15 mM EDTA, 1.2mM dithiothreitol and 10% glycerol).

When the tissue was converted to a turbid mixture, then it was filtered through several layers of nylon gauze to eliminate fibers and connective tissue. The filtrate was centrifuged at 1600xg for 20min at $4^0$C in order to get rid of all the remaining intact cells and nuclei. The supernatant was stored at $-20^0$C till the time for use.

## 2.6. Estimation of Protein Contents:

Protein was measured by the method of Lowry *et al.*,[128]. Using BSA as standard.

## 2.7. Determinations of Total PSA in Sera of Patients and Controls:

### Reagents:

1- Monoclonal $^{125}$I-anti total PSA antibody in vial contains less than 580KBq with protein, buffer, sodium azide and a dye.

2- Five vials of standards contained the concentrations 0, 0.9, 2.7, 9, 27, 90 ng. ml$^{-1}$ of prostate specific antigen.

3- Anti PSA monoclonal antibody coated tubes. The inner surface of each tube is coated with antibody directed against one of PSA epitopes.

4- Lyophilized control sera. Human serum and preservative.

5- Washing solution.

## Procedure:

1- From each standard or sample a 100µl was pipetted to an antibody coated tube.

2- From the tracer (reagent No.1) 100µl were added to each tube and the content of the tube was vortexed.

3- Two tubes were prepared separately for total radioactivity (T) measurements and contained 100µl of tracer.

4- The tubes were incubated for two hours at room temperature (18-25$^0$C) with shaking.

5- The contents of all the tubes except those for total radioactivity was aspirated thoroughly.

6- The tubes were washed with 2ml of washing solution (with exception of those for T measurements). This step was repeated twice and all the remains of the fluids were disposed.

7- All the tubes were measured for 1min in gamma counter to determine the radioactivity of each tube.

## *Calculations:*

1- The gamma counter records the net count of the radioactivity of the tube within 1min.

2- The radioactivity of each tube refers to the amount of bound PSA to the inner surface of the coated tube and represented by B.

3- The B/T% was calculated where

$$B/T\% = \frac{\text{Standard or sample C.P.M}}{\text{Total radioactivity C.P.M}} \times 100$$

4- Standard curve was constructed by plotting B/T% against corresponding PSA standard concentration in log-log coordinate as in figure (2-1).

5- The unknown concentrations of samples were obtained from the equation of the straight line of the standard curve.

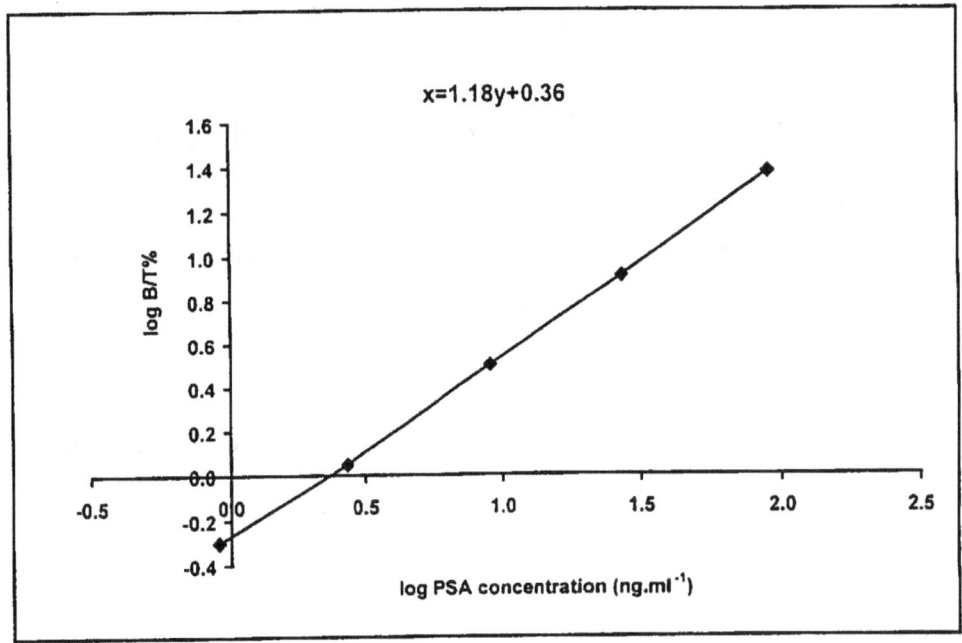

*Figure (2-1): Standard curve of total PSA measurements*

*All other details are explained in the text*

## 2.8. Determinations of Total PSA in Benign and Malignant Prostate Tissue

The IRMA was capable to measure PSA levels in serum and in order to be applicable for determination of PSA in tissue, a standard additions method was performed to ensure that there is no interference if tissue was in use and the IRMA was capable to determine PSA levels in tissue with high accuracy.

### Recovery determination

1- To a coated tubes 100µl (50µg protein) of Prostate cancer tissue homogenate was transferred.

2- Hundred micro liter of standard PSA containing the concentrations (0, 5.4, 18, 54, 72ng.ml$^{-1}$) was added and vortexed for a while.

3- PSA level in each tube was determined as mentioned in section 2.2.8.

4- The obtained actual concentration was compared with the expected values as in table (2-1).

*Table (2-1): The Standard Additions Method of the Determination of PSA in Prostate Cancer Tissue by IRMA. (Recovery determination)*

| Tube No. | Homogenate volume µl | Standard Conc. ng.ml$^{-1}$ | C.P.M | Actual PSA Conc. ng.ml$^{-1}$ | Expected PSA Conc. ng.ml$^{-1}$ | Recovery % |
|---|---|---|---|---|---|---|
| 1 | 100 | 0 | 557 | 7.24 | - | - |
| 2 | 100 | 5.4 | 699 | 9.55 | 9.94 | 96 |
| 3 | 100 | 18 | 1163 | 16.79 | 16.24 | 103 |
| 4 | 100 | 54 | 2083 | 34.67 | 34.24 | 101 |
| 5 | 100 | 72 | 2566 | 44.64 | 43.24 | 103 |

The comparison of actual and expected PSA concentrations and the recovery values reveals that the interferences of homogenate proteins could be negligible. Accordingly the measurements of PSA concentrations in homogenate was performed as mentioned in serum PSA determination in section 2.7.

## 2.9. Determination of PSA Density (PSAD):

Prostate specific antigen density (PSAD) was obtained by dividing the concentration of PSA (ng.ml$^{-1}$) by the volume of the prostate gland in milliliter (ml). TRUS gives the diameter of each dimension of prostate gland d1, d2, d3 in cm. These dimensions can be transformed into volume according to the following equation[129].

Volume = 0.52 × d1 × d2 × d3

$$PSAD = \frac{PSA\ Conc.\ (ng.ml^{-1})}{Volume\ (ml)}$$

## 2.10. Binding Studies of Prostate Specific Antigen in Prostate Cancer Tissue and([125]I-Anti Total PSA Antibody).

### 2.10.1. Preliminary Test of the Binding of PSA of Prostate Cancer Tissue with ([125]I-Anti Total PSA Antibody).

1- A volume of 50μl(25μg protein) of prostate cancer tissue homogenate was incubated with 50μl (225μg protein) of [125]I-anti total PSA antibody at room temperature (about 20⁰C) for 2hours with continuous shaking.

2- The volume was completed to 300µl with tris buffer pH7.4.

3- Two tubes contained 50µl of $^{125}$I-anti total PSA antibody only for total activity computation.

4- The tubes were centrifuged immediately at 1500xg in a cooling centrifuge for 20min.

5- The supernatant was removed by gentle decantation and the pellets were washed with 200µl of buffer then the tubes were inverted on a dry filter paper for 10min.

6- The rims of the tube were swabbed with a cotton and the radioactivity was measured by gamma counter in addition to the tubes of the total radio activity.

## Calculations:

1- The radioactivity of the tube in count per minute (CPM) represents the amount of the formed complex (antigen-antibody) and denoted by the symbol B.

2- The radioactivity of the tubes that contained only the tracer represent the total radioactivity T.

3- The ratio B/T% was calculated as follow.

$$B/T\% = \frac{\text{Sample count B(CPM)}}{\text{Total radioactivity T(CPM)}} \times 100$$

## 2.10.2. Most Appropriate Conditions of Binding of Prostate Specific Antigen in Prostate Cancer Tissue with ($^{125}$I Anti Total PSA Antibody)

### 2.10.2.1. The Effect of Different concentrations of($^{125}$I-Anti Total PSA Antibody)on the Binding with Prostate Specific Antigen in Prostate Cancer Tissue.

1- The volumes of 6,12,18,24,36,48,60µl of $^{125}$I-anti total PSA antibody containing 27,54,81,108,162,216,270µl of protein respectively, where each added to a 50µl (25mg protein) of prostate cancer tissue homogenate. The volumes completed with tris buffer pH7.4 to 300µl.

2- Other two tubes containing only 60µl (270µg protein) of $^{125}$I-anti total PSA antibody where set aside for total radioactivity computation.

3- All tubes were closed with parafilm tightly and incubated for 2hours at room temp with continuous shaking.

4- After incubation time, the tubes were centrifuged for 20min at 4$^0$C to precipitate the formed complex (antigen-antibody)

5- The supernatant was decanted gently, and the pellet was washed with 200µl of tris buffer PH7.4, then the tubes were inverted on a filter paper for 10min.

6- The rims of the tubes were swabbed with cotton and the radioactivity was counted in the gamma counter.

## *Calculations:*

1- The measured radioactivity was denoted by the symbol B and represents the bound part of PSA.

2- The total radioactivity T was obtained from the total radioactivity measurement in CPM.

3- The B/T% was obtained as follow

$$B/T\% = \frac{CPM \text{ of the tube (B)}}{CPM \text{ of total radioactivity (T)}} \times 100$$

4- The B/T% values were plotted against the concentrations of tracer.

### 2.10.2.2. The Effect of Different Protein Concentrations of Prostate Cancer Tissue on the Binding of Prostate Specific Antigen with ($^{125}$I-Anti Total PSA Antibody):

1- The volumes (5,10,15,25,50,75,100µl) of prostate cancer tissue homogenate containing(2.5, 5, 7.5, 12.5, 25, 37.5 µg of protein) respectively, were added to 24µl (108µg of protein).

2- Tubes volume were made up to 300µl with tris buffer pH 7.4 and two other tubes were contained only 24µl of $^{125}$I-anti total PSA antibody for total activity computation.

3- The tubes were incubated for 2hours at room temperature with continuous shaking.

4- After the incubation time, the tubes were centrifuged for 20min and the supernatant was disposed.

5- The radioactivity of the tubes were measured in addition to the total radioactivity.

## Calculations:

1- B/T% was calculated as mentioned in sec. 2.10.1.

2- B/T% was plotted versus protein concentration of prostate cancer tissue homogenate.

### 2.10.2.3. *The Effect of pH on the Binding of Prostate Specific Antigen of Prostate Cancer Tissue with($^{125}$I-Anti Total PSA Antibody).*

1- Different tris buffers pH (7,7.2,7.4,7.6,7.8,8) were prepared.

2- Volume of 50μl (25μg protein) of prostate cancer tissue homogenate was added to 24μl (108μg protein) of $^{125}$I-anti total PSA antibody. The total volume was made up to 300μl by one of the tris buffers that mentioned in step1.

3- Two additional tubes containing 24μl of $^{125}$I-anti total PSA antibody were set aside for total radioactivity computation.

4- After two hours of incubation, the tubes were centrifuged for 20min and the supernatant were decanted.

5- The radioactivity of all the tubes were measured by gamma counter, as well as the other two tubes for total radioactivity determination.

### *Calculations:*

1- B/T% was calculated as mentioned in section 2.10.1.

2- B/T% was plotted against the corresponding pH values.

### 2.10.2.4. *The Effect of Temperature on the Binding of Prostate Specific Antigen of Prostate Cancer Tissue with ($^{125}$I-Anti Total PSA Antibody).*

1- A volume of 24μl (108μg protein) of $^{125}$I-anti total PSA antibody was added to 50μl (25μg protein) of prostate cancer tissue homogenate. The volume was made up to 300μl with tris buffer pH7.2.

2- The tubes were incubated for two hours at different temperatures (4,20,37,45$^0$C).

3- Two additional tubes contained only 24µl of $^{125}$I-anti total PSA antibody were set aside for total radioactivity computation.

4- After two hours of incubation, the tubes were centrifuged for 20min and the supernatants were decanted.

5- The radioactivity of all the tubes were measured including the tubes for total radioactivity.

*Calculations:*

1- B/T% was calculated as mentioned in section 2.10.1.

2- B/T% was constructed versus temperature points.

### 2.10.2.5. Optimum Incubation Time for the Binding of Prostate Specific Antigen of Prostate Cancer Tissue with ($^{125}$I-Anti Total PSA Antibody).

1- A volume of 24µl (108µg Protein) of $^{125}$I-anti total PSA antibody was added to 50µl (25µg protein) of prostate cancer tissue homogenate. The volume was made up to 300µl with tris buffer pH7.2.

2- Two additional tubes were occupied with 24µl of $^{125}$I-anti total PSA antibody only and set aside for total radioactivity computation.

3- The tubes (except those for total radioactivity) were incubated for different intervals of times (15,30,60,90,120,150,180 and 240min)at 45$^0$C.

4- After the incubation time of each tube. Each tube was centrifuged and the supernatant was decanted.

6- The radioactivity of each tube was measured by gamma counter in addition to those tubes of total radioactivity.

## Calculations:

1- B/T% was calculated as mentioned in section 2.10.1.

2- B/T% was plotted versus the time of incubation in minutes.

### 2.10.2.6. The Effect of Different Halides on the Binding of Prostate Specific Antigen of Prostate Cancer Tissue with ($^{125}$I-Anti Total PSA Antibody).

1- A volume of 50μl (25μg protein) of prostate cancer tissue homogenate was added to 20μl (108μg protein) of $^{125}$I-anti total PSA antibody, the volume was completed to 300μl with salty tris buffer pH7.2 table (2-2) shows the preparation of salty tris buffer pH7.2.

2- The incubation was performed at 45$^0$C for two hours.

3- Two additional tubes contained only 24μl of $^{125}$I-anti total PSA antibody were set aside for total radioactivity computation.

*Table (2-2): The Weights of the Added Halide Salts to 10ml of Tris Buffer pH7.2.*

| Sodium Halides \ Molar Concentration | 0.05 | 0.1 | 0.2 | 0.4 |
|---|---|---|---|---|
| F | 26.5 | 53.0 | 106.0 | 212.1 |
| Cl | 37.8 | 75.0 | 151.1 | 302.2 |
| Br | 66.6 | 133.7 | 266.3 | 532.7 |
| I | 96.9 | 193.8 | 387.6 | 775.3 |

**Note:** All salts weight in mg.

4- After incubation the tubes were centrifuged and the supernatants were decanted.

5- The radioactivity of each tube was measured in addition to those two tubes for total radioactivity determination.

## *Calculations:*

1- B/T% was determined to each tube as mentioned in section 2.10.1.

2- B/T% was plotted against the concentration of each salt.

**2.10.2.7. The Effect of Divalent Cations on the Binding of Prostate Specific Antigen of Prostate Cancer Tissue with ($^{125}$I-Anti Total PSA Antibody).**

1- A volume of 24µl (108µg protein) of $^{125}$I-anti total PSA antibody, was added to 50µl(25µg protein) of prostate cancer tissue homogenate. The volume was completed to 300µl with salty tris buffer pH7.2 table (2-3) shows the contents of the salty tris buffer. pH7.2.

2- The incubation was performed at 45 $^0$C for two hours.

3- Two additional tubes were contained only 24µl of $^{125}$I-anti total PSA antibody were set aside for total radioactivity computation.

*Table (2-3):The Weight of the Added Divalent Salts to 10ml of Tris Buffer pH7.2*

| Molar concentration / Chloride Salts | 0.005 | 0.01 | 0.025 | 0.05 | 0.1 |
|---|---|---|---|---|---|
| Mg | 6.2 | 12.3 | 30.8 | 61.5 | 123.3 |
| Ca | 7.2 | 14.3 | 35.8 | 71.7 | 143.4 |
| Zn | 8.8 | 17.6 | 44.0 | 88.0 | 176.1 |

**Note:** All divalent salts weight in mg.

4- After incubation, the tubes were centrifuged and the supernatants were decanted.

5- The radioactivity of each tube was measured in addition to those two tubes for total radioactivity determination.

## Calculations:

1- B/T% was determined to each tube as mentioned in section 2.10.1.

2- B/T% was plotted against the concentration of each salt.

### 2.10.2.8. The Effect of Polyethylene Glycol on the Binding of Prostate Specific Antigen of Prostate Cancer Tissue with ($^{125}$I-Anti Total PSA Antibody).

1- A volume of 24μl (108μg protein) of $^{125}$I-anti total PSA antibody, was added to 50μl(25μg protein) of prostate cancer tissue homogenate. The volume was completed to 300μl with tris buffer pH7.2. (contained in each time one of the following percents of polyethylene glycol 0.66, 1.33, 3.32, 6.64, 13.27% weight to volume) to 300μl as a final volume.

2- Two additional tubes contained only 24μl of $^{125}$I-anti total PSA antibody.

3- The tubes were incubated for two hours at $45^0$C.

4- After incubation the tubes (except those for total radioactivity) were centrifuged and the supernatants were decanted.

6- The radioactivity of each tube was measured in addition to those two tubes for total radioactivity computation.

## Calculations:

1- B/T% was determined at each tube as mentioned in section 2.10.1.

2- B/T% was plotted against the percent of polyethylene glycol.

## 2.11. Kinetics Studies on the Reaction Between Prostate Specific Antigen of Prostate Cancer Tissue and ($^{125}$I-Anti Total PSA Antibody).

### 2.11.1. .Determination of Affinity Constant and Maximal Binding Capacity of the reaction Between Prostate Specific Antigen of Prostate Cancer Tissue and ($^{125}$I-Anti Total PSA Antibody).

1- A volume of 50μl (25μg protein) of prostate cancer tissue homogenate was added to each of the volumes 6,12,18,24μl of $^{125}$I-anti total PSA antibody contained (27, 54, 81, 108μg protein) respectively.

2- The volume were completed to 300μl with tris buffer pH7.2.

3- The tubes were incubated at 45$^0$C for two hours.

4- The steps 1,2,3 were repeated with different temperatures 4,20,37$^0$C.

5- After incubation time the radioactivity of each tube was determined then the tubes were centrifuged and the supernatants were decanted.

6- The radioactivity of each tube was determined by gamma counter.

## *Calculations:*

1- B/T was determined for each tube as mentioned in section 2.10.1

2- B/F was calculated from B/T value as follow.

F : The free radioactivity which represents the free part of $^{125}$I-anti total PSA antibody.

$$\frac{F}{B} = \frac{T-B}{B}$$

$$\frac{B}{F} = \frac{B}{T-B} \;.$$

3- The concentration of the formed complex (B) was calculated as follow

$$B \text{ (mg.ml}^{-1}) = \frac{B(c.p.m.)}{T(c.p.m)} \;.\; \text{concentration of tracer in the incubation media in mg.ml}^{-1}.$$

4- The affinity constant (Ka) and maximal binding capacity (Bmax) were determined according to Scatchard equation.

$$\frac{B}{F} = Ka \,(B \max - B)$$

5- The dissociation constant Kd was also determined as follow

$$Kd = \frac{1}{Ka}$$

6- The plot of B/F versus (B) may construct a linear relationship. The slop of the straight line represents Ka while the intercept of the straight-line with (x)axis refers to (Bmax) value.

## 2.11.2 The Time Course of the Binding of Prostate Cancer Tissue with ($^{125}$I-Anti Total PSA Antibody).

1- A volume of 24μl (108μg protein) of $^{125}$I-anti total PSA antibody was added to 50μl(25μg protein) of prostate cancer tissue homogenate. The volume was made up to 300μl with tris buffer pH7.2.

2- Other additional two tubes contained only 24μl of $^{125}$I-anti total PSA antibody were set aside for total radioactivity computation.

3- The tubes were incubated at $45^0C$ for different intervals of times 15,30,60,90,20,50,80,210,240 minutes.

4- The steps 1,2,3 were repeated with temperatures $4,20,37^0C$.

5- After incubation time the tubes were centrifuged and the supernatants were decanted.

6- The radioactivity of all the tubes were measured by gamma counter in addition to those two for total radioactivity computation.

## *Calculations:*

1- B/T% was determined for each tube as mentioned in section 2.10.1.

2- B/T% was plotted against intervals of incubation.

## 2.12. Thermodynamics Studies on the Reaction Between Prostate Specific Antigen of Prostate Cancer Tissue and ($^{125}$I-Anti Total PSA Antibody).

### 2.12.1. Standard State:

The thermodynamic parameters of standard state ($\Delta H^0$, $\Delta G^0$, $\Delta S^0$) were obtained from Vant Hoff plot. The values of the natural logarithm of equilibrium constant (affinity constant Ka) which obtained at different temperatures were plotted against the reciprocal values of absolute temperature in Kelvin (1/T) and $\Delta H$ value was calculated from the slope of the following equation of Vant Hoff.

$$Ln\ Ka = \frac{\Delta S^0}{R} - \frac{\Delta H^0}{RT}$$

Where

$\Delta H^0$ : The enthalpy change at standard state.

$\Delta S^0$ : The entropy change at standard state.

R   : Gas constant (8.314 J.K$^{-1}$.mol$^{-1}$).

T   : Temperature in Kelvin.

The change in Gibbs free energy of the standard state $\Delta G^0$ was obtained from the following equation.

$$\Delta G^0 = -RT \ln ka$$

While the entropy change in the standards state was obtained from Gibbs equation.

$$\Delta S^0 = \frac{\Delta H^0 - \Delta G^0}{T}$$

### 2.12.2 Transition State:

Initially the thermodynamic parameters of the transition state were obtained from Arrhenius equation by plotting $\ln K_{+1}$ values against 1/T values. The given linear relationship was obtained according to the following equation.

$$\ln K_{+1} = \ln A - \left( \frac{Ea}{RT} \right)$$

Where

A: Arrhenius constant.

Ea : Energy of activation

T  : Absolute temperature in Kelvin

The  value of Ea of the binding reaction can be determined from the slope of the straight line.

The enthalpy change of the transition state $\Delta H^*$ was obtained from the equation

$$\Delta H^* = Ea - RT$$

The free energy change of transition state $\Delta G^*$ was calculated using the following equation.

$$\Delta G^* = -RT \ln K_{+1} + RT \ln\left(\frac{KT}{h}\right)$$

Where

$K$ : Boltzmann constant : $1.38 \times 10^{-23}$ J.deg$^{-1}$

$h$ : Plank constant : $0.662 \times 10^{-33}$ J.S$^{-1}$

The change in the entropy of the transition state ($\Delta S^*$) was calculated from the following equation:

$$\Delta S^* = \frac{\Delta H^* - \Delta G^*}{T}$$

# 3. Results and Discussion:

## 3.1. Prostate Specific Antigen Levels in Sera of Patients with Prostate Cancer and Benign Prostatic Hyperplasia

Prostate specific antigen (PSA) levels were determined using the radioimmunometric assay (IRMA), in patients with different stages of prostate cancer and benign prostatic hyperplasia. The results were compared with PSA levels in age matched controls. Table (2-4) shows these results with age ranges of those individuals.

*Table (2-4): Prostate Specific Antigen Levels in Sera of Patients with Prostate Cancer and Benign Prostatic Hyperplasia*

| CASE | No. | AGE Years | PSA ng.ml$^{-1}$ | | |
|------|-----|-----------|---|----|-----|
| | | | X | SD | CV% |
| Prostate cancer | 36 | 47-80 | 50.8 | 111.6 | 219.6 |
| BPH | 52 | 45-80 | 7.1 | 3.2 | 45.1 |
| Control | 41 | 45-75 | 2.3 | 0.8 | 34.8 |

In table (2-4) the control mean of PSA level was 2.3 ng.ml$^{-1}$ which represents the normal value of prostate specific antigen in those Iraqi people. It was less than the cut-off value (4 ng.ml$^{-1}$) of PSA. The former value was considered by many investigators as the border line between normal and abnormal prostate status[130,131]. The mean of PSA concentration of prostate cancer was 50.8 ng.ml$^{-1}$. While that for BPH was 7.1 ng.ml$^{-1}$, hence there is a significant difference (P>0.05) between the two values. In spite of the significant difference between the two means, the distinction between prostate cancer and benign prostate hyperplasia was insufficient specially at the range 4-10ng.ml$^{-1}$ where the overlaping between the two ranges was in maximum[132]. The highly overlaping may make the outcome of PSA test less effective for making prostate cancer diagnosis [133]. Particularly when the low sensitivity (57-70%) and specificity (59-68%) of PSA was considered[134].

## 3.2. Prostate Specific Antigen Density in Prostate Cancer and Benign Prostatic Hyperplasia.

Prostate specific antigen density (PSAD) was introduced as a method by which the ratio of serum PSA and prostate volume could be used to improve the ability to differentiate between prostate cancer and benign prostatic hyperplasia[135]. Table (2-5) shows that PSAD level in prostate cancer was 0.81 ng.ml$^{-1}$/ml and it was 0.14 ng.ml$^{-1}$/ml in patients with BPH. There was a significant difference (P>0.05) between the two means.

*Table (2-5): Prostate Specific Antigen Density in Prostate Cancer and Benign Prostatic Hyperplasia.*

| Case | No | Age year | Prostate Volume(ml) | | PSA ng.ml$^{-1}$ | | PSAD ng.ml$^{-1}$/ml | |
|---|---|---|---|---|---|---|---|---|
| | | | X | SD | X | SD | X | SD |
| Prostate cancer | 25 | 47-80 | 49.2 | 27.3 | 50.2 | 95.7 | 0.81 | 0.92 |
| Benign Prostatic hyperplasia | 32 | 45-80 | 52.8 | 26.1 | 7.3 | 3.1 | 0.14 | 0.73 |

The cut-off value of PSAD is 0.15 ng.ml$^{-1}$/ml. Based on this value a serial tests of PSA would be advised for aged men with a PSAD of 0.15ng.ml$^{-1}$/ml or less but, for patients with a normal DRE and PSAD above 0.15ng.ml$^{-1}$/ml abiopsy would be recommended.[135]. Its obvious from our results of PSAD that prostate cancer tissue secrete or leaks more PSA to the circulation than prostate tissue of BPH. This result was in consistant with the speculation of Stamey *et al*[136] who mentioned that prostate cancer leaks 10 times more PSA into blood stream than does benign hyperplastic tissue. Accordingly a high PSAD is more likely to be caused by prostate cancer.

## 3.3. Postoperative Level of Prostate Specific Antigen in Prostate Cancer.

Figure (2-2) displays the weekly decline in postoperative serum PSA levels in three patients with prostate cancer.

PSA level had increased at first weeks after surgery. The enhancement of PSA exceeded the preoperative value of PSA, accordingly, postoperative PSA value was not reflected the expected values in this period of time and therefore PSA level at first three weeks after surgery would not serve as a monitoring tool for prostatic status so that the clinical importance of PSA in evaluating outcome after operations would be reduced to large extent. This results were corroborated by Frazier *et al*[137] finding in their study on sera PSA level for clinically localized prostate cancer. They observed that the patients had and elevated serum PSA values one month after surgery. However, figure (2-2), also displays the postoperative PSA levels with time.

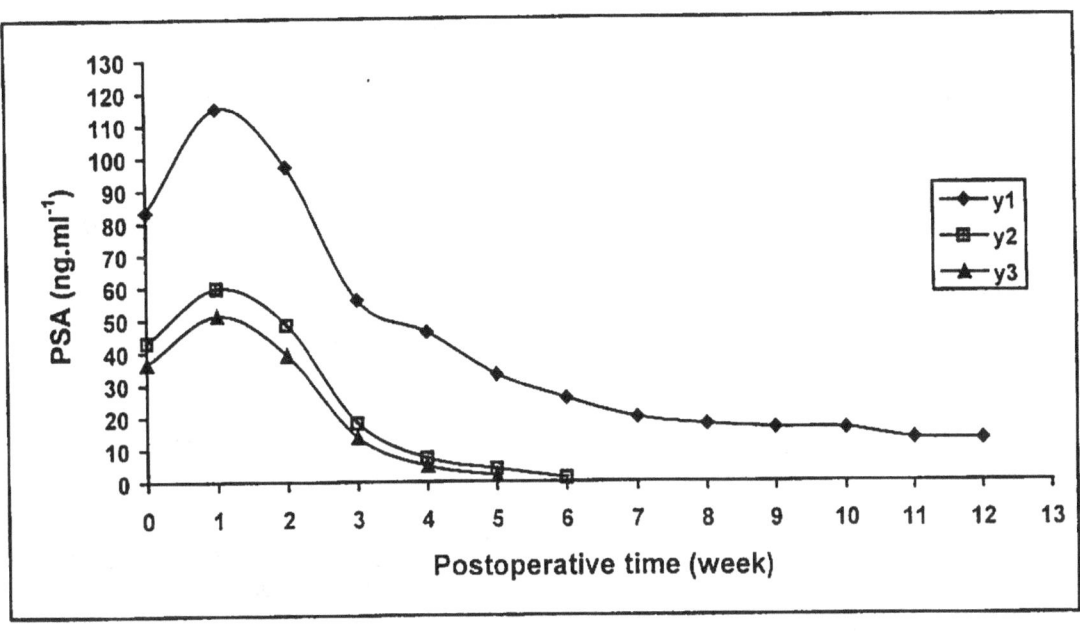

*Figure (2-2): The postoperative levels of prostate specific antigen in prostate*

*cancer. All other details are explained in the text.*

The decrement especially at first three weeks was not well correlated with the half-life of PSA in the circulation. The half-life of PSA was frequently reported by many investigators. It was approximately 3.15days[138] or 4.2 days[139], so that, by using the aforementioned calculated half-life serum PSA level of 50ng.ml$^{-1}$ should be undetectable 30days after curative radical prostatectomy[140]. Tissue damage during the operation may be responsible for this phenomenon but the detectable serum PSA levels following surgery was attributed by Portin *et al*[141] either to local recurrence or to distant metastases subsequently developed.

## 3.4. Prostate Specific Antigen in Tissue of Prostate Cancer and Benign Prostatic Hyperplasia.

PSA concentration was determined in prostate cancer and in benign prostatic hyperplasia tissues by immuno radiometric assay. The results in table (2-6) revealed that the mean of PSA levels in prostate cancer tissue was 7.41 mg.g$^{-1}$(protein) and its significantly (P<0.05) higher than that of benign prostatic hyperplasia which was 4.37 mg.g$^{-1}$ (protein).

*Table (2-6): Prostate Specific Antigen Levels in Prostate Cancer and Benign Prostatic Hyperplasia.*

| CASE | No. | AGE Years | PSA mg.g$^{-1}$ (protein) | | |
|---|---|---|---|---|---|
| | | | X | SD | CV% |
| Prostate cancer (cancerous tissue) | 21 | 47-80 | 7.41 | 3.3 | 44.6 |
| Prostate cancer (non-cancerous tissue) | 21 | 47-80 | 9.73 | 4.7 | 48.3 |
| BPH | 31 | 45-75 | 4.37 | 1.8 | 41.1 |

The enhancement of PSA in prostate cancer tissue may attributed to the raise in expression of PSA gene. The expression of PSA gene is under complex control and the steady-state level of PSA, mRNA is increased by androgens, and decreased by epidermal growth factor[142] but the real cause of enhancement of PSA expression in malignant tissues of prostate cancer is still obscure. Etsuo *et al.,*[143] reported that the precise significance of elevated PSA in prostate cancer remains unknown. In table (2-6) PSA level in non- cancerous tissue of prostate was significantly higher than PSA level in cancerous tissue (they both were obtained from the same patients). This result may suggests that the PSA may play a role in the defense mechanism against cancer. The higher secretion of PSA from non cancerous tissue may be stimulated by the invasive effect of the nearby malignant cells. The decrement in PSA level in malignant tissue compared with benign prostatic tissue was also reported by David *et al*[144] who mentioned that cancer producers less PSA per cell than benign epithelium. The idea of PSA to be a means of defence or protection against cancer was first produced by Eleftherios *et al*[145] Who mentioned that PSA should be considered as a ((cancer fighter) at the tissue level and as a valuable messenger (indicator) at the level of systematic circulation. It has been thus suggested that effort to produce cancer vaccines or other therapies targeting PSA expression may be the wrong strategy and that treatment approaches to treat prostate and possibly breast, cancer should be directed toward over expression of PSA at the tissue levels[146,147].

## 3.5. Binding Studies on Prostate Specific Antigen of Prostate Cancer with ([125]I-Anti Total PSA Antibody).

### 3.5.1. Preliminary Test of the Binding of Prostate Specific Antigen of Prostate Cancer with ([125]I-Anti Total PSA Antibody).

The prostate specific antigen which was obtained from homogenization of prostate cancer tissue reacts as an antigen when incubated with [125]I-anti total PSA antibody for 2hours to form a separate complex by centrifugation at 1500xg. The high molecular weight complex was precipitated and accumulated in the bottom of the tube to form small pellets. The preliminary conditions used in this experiment resulted in 3.9% binding.

## 3.5.2. Most Appropriate Conditions of the Binding of Prostate Specific Antigen of Prostate Cancer Tissue with ($^{125}$I-Anti Total PSA Antibody)

### 3.5.2.1. The Effect of Different Concentrations of Prostate Specific Antigen of Prostate Cancer Tissue on the Binding with ($^{125}$I-Anti Total PSA Antibody)

Complex formation depends to large extent on the concentration of $^{125}$I-Anti total PSA Antibody. The experiment for determination of the optimum tracer concentration was designed to proceed while other conditions were stable except the concentration of $^{125}$I-anti total PSA antibody which was variable in a range that enable to determine the optimum point of tracer concentration. Figure(2-3) shows that the optimum tracer concentration was 0.36mg.ml$^{-1}$.

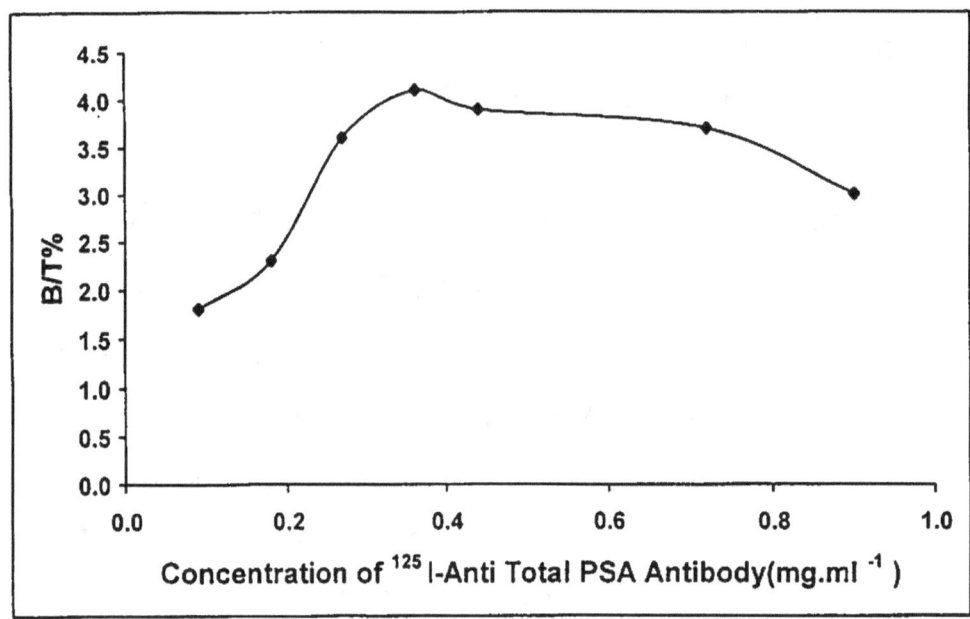

*Figure (2-3): The optimum concentration of $^{125}$I anti total PSA antibody in the reaction with prostate specific antigen of prostate cancer tissue. All other details are explained in the text.*

### 3.5.2.2. The Effect of Different Concentrations of Prostate Specific Antigen of Prostate Cancer Tissue on the Binding with ($^{125}$I-Anti Total PSA Antibody)

The alteration in the concentration of PSA of prostate cancer tissue influence the binding of this antigen to its specific antibody. To explore this fact practically, a set of increased concentration of homogenate was prepared while the tracer and all other experimental condition still fixed through out the experiment.

Figure (2-4) displays the changes of binding percent that occur with the enhancement of PSA levels. The optimum binding was at concentration 0.083mg.ml$^{-1}$ of homogenate protein.

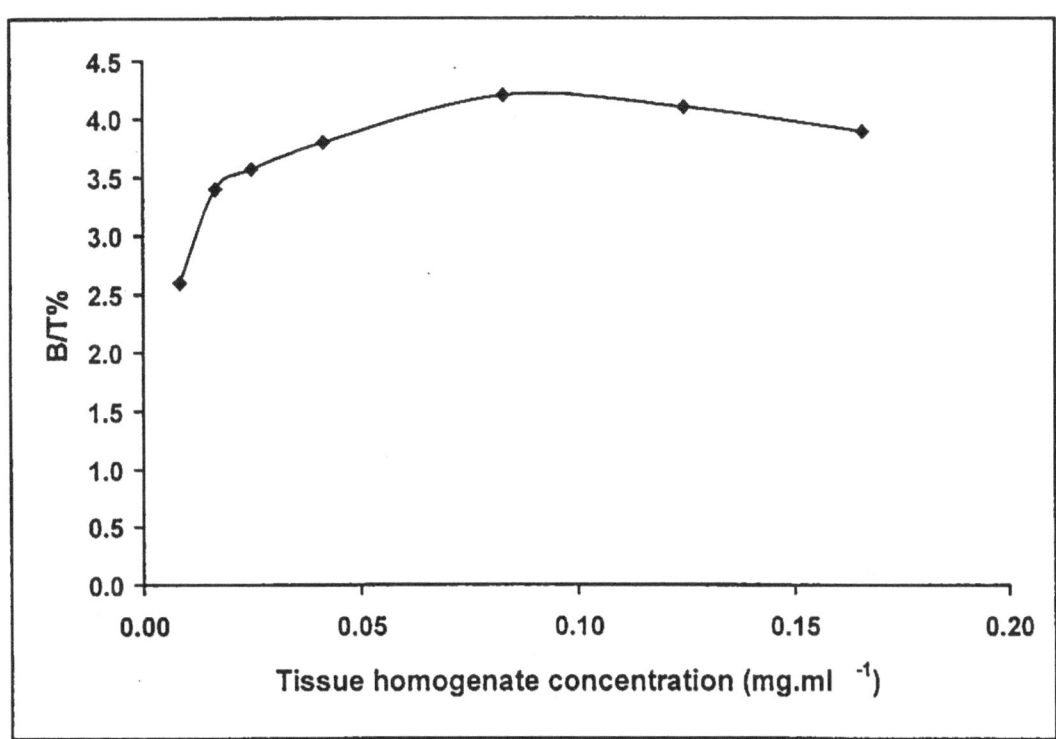

*Figure (2-4): The optimum concentration of prostate specific antigen of prostate cancer tissue in the reaction with ($^{125}$I-anti total PSA antibody). All other details are explained in the text.*

### 3.5.2.3. The Effect of Different pH on the Binding of Prostate Specific Antigen of Prostate Cancer and ($^{125}$I-Anti Total PSA Antibody)

The effect of pH changes on the tendency of PSA of prostate cancer tissue homogenate to associate with $^{125}$I-anti total PSA antibody was examined.

Figure (2-5) illustrate the relationship between pH and the binding percent. The highest binding percent was achieved at pH 7.2. This result may either indicate that the immunoreactivity of the reactants or the stability of the formed complex enhanced at certain point of pH[148] therefore all next experiments were carried out at pH7.2.

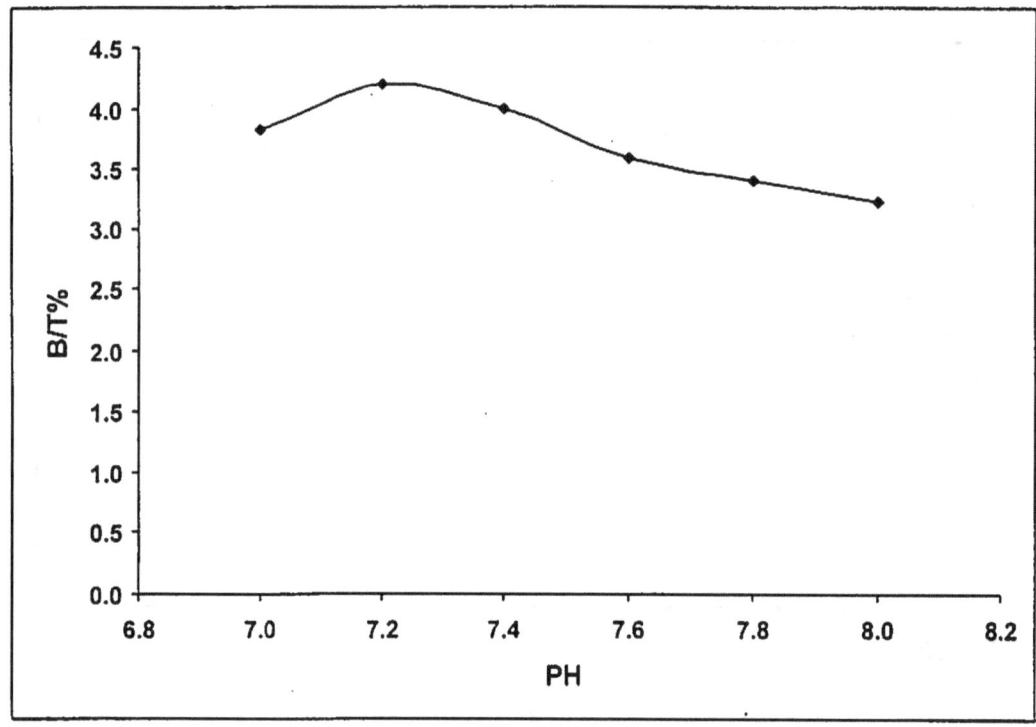

*Figure (2-5): Optimum pH for the binding of prostate specific antigen of prostate cancer with ($^{125}$I-anti total PSA antibody). All other details are explained in the text.*

### 3.5.2.4. The Effect of the Temperature on the Binding of Prostate Specific Antigen of Prostate Cancer with($^{125}$I-Anti Total PSA Antibody)

This investigation also include the temperature dependency of the binding between prostate specific antigen of prostate cancer tissue and $^{125}$I-anti total PSA antibody. In figure (2-6) four points of temperature were selected for the determination of binding percent of the antigen-antibody reaction. The binding percent was enhanced with temperature raise so that the most appropriate temperature for binding was $45^0$C and therefore all next experiments were carried out at this temperature.

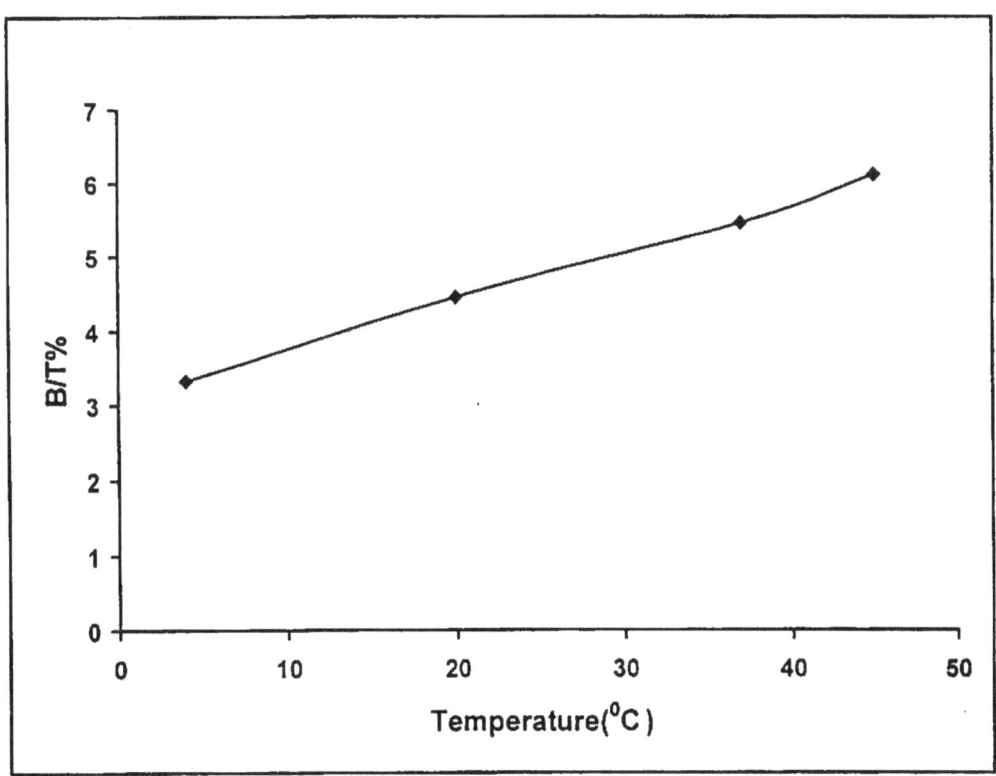

*Figure (2-6):Optimum temperature for the binding of prostate specific antigen of prostate cancer with ($^{125}$I-anti total PSA antibody). All other details are explained in the text.*

### 3.5.2.5. The Most Appropriate Incubation Time for Binding of Prostate Specific Antigen of Prostate Cancer with ($^{125}$I-Anti Total PSA Antibody)

The reaction between prostate specific antigen of prostate cancer tissue homogenate and $^{125}$I-anti total PSA antibody is a time dependent process. Figure (2-7) displays the alteration in binding percent with change in incubation times at temperature $45^0$C. The optimum time was 120min, at this time the highest binding percent was met. Accordingly, the incubation time in all subsequent experiment was 120min.

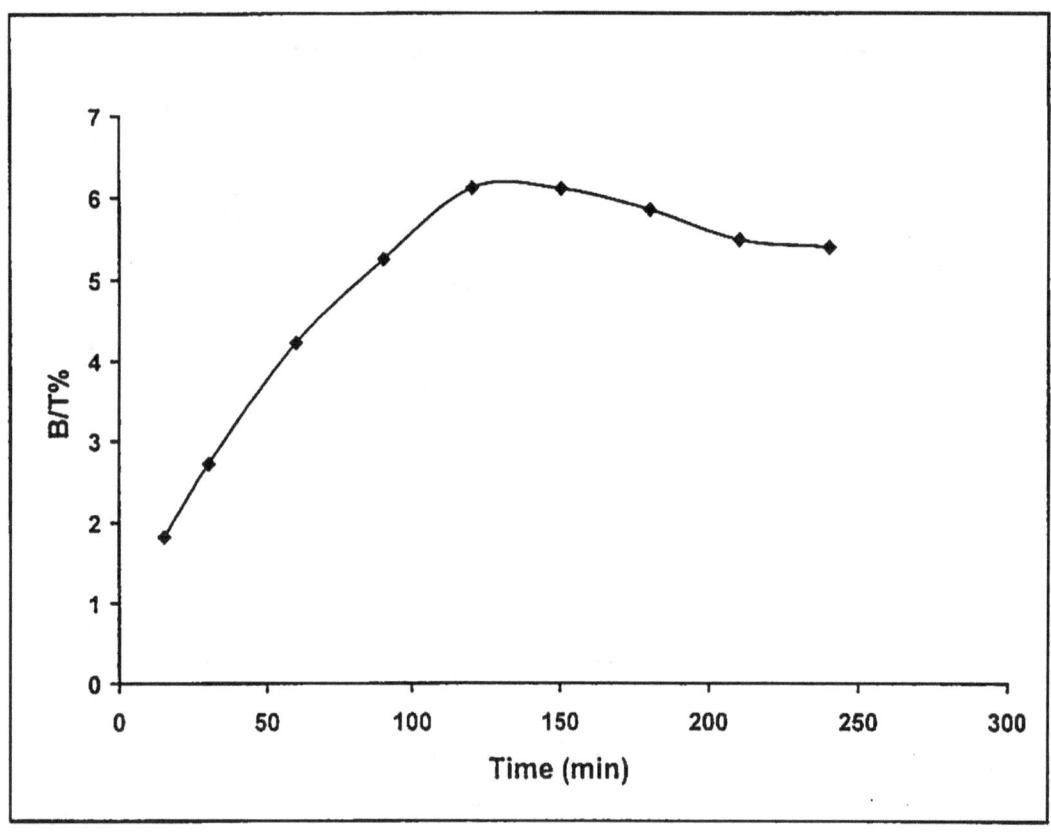

*Figure (2-7):Time course of the binding of prostate specific antigen of prostate cancer with ($^{125}$I-anti total PSA antibody). All other details are explained in the text.*

### 3.5.2.6 *The Effect Different Halides on the Binding of Prostate Specific Antigen of Prostate Cancer with ($^{125}$I-Anti Total PSA Antibody)*

The halides F,Cl,Br,I, all were investigated to estimate its effect on the binding process to form a complex between prostate specific antigen of prostate cancer tissue homogenate and $^{125}$I-anti total PSA antibody. Figure (2-8) shows the selected concentrations of halides and the relative binding percents. Its clear that there is a general trend to decline in binding percent with increasing ionic strength of incubation media with exception of the iodide where the binding percent seems to be constant with the raise of molar concentration.

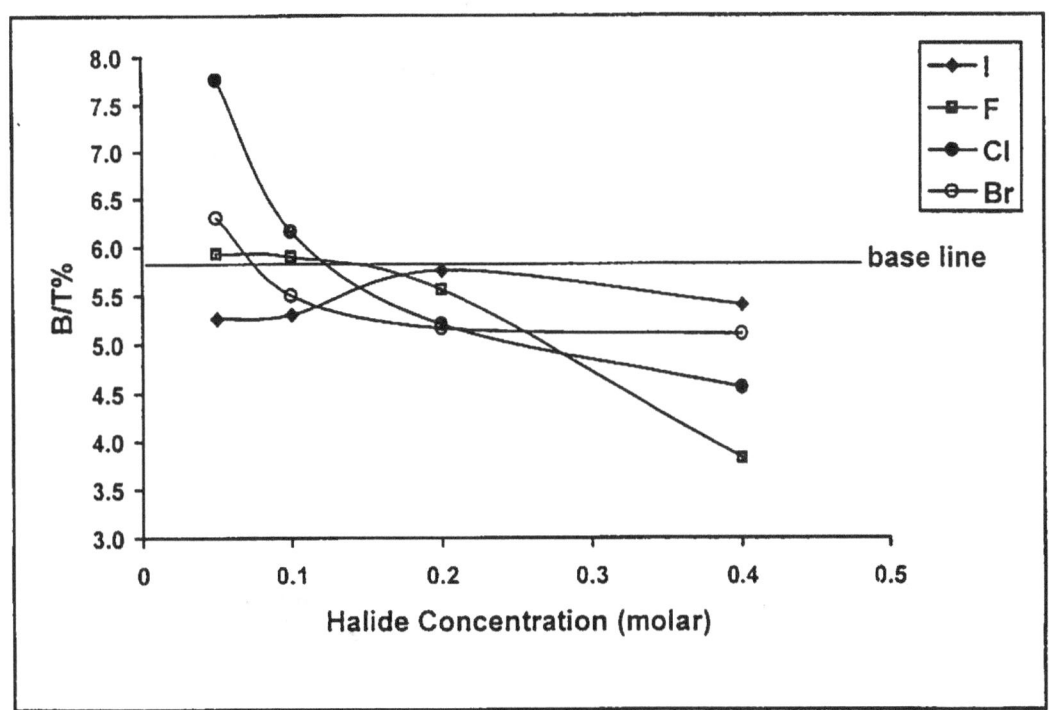

*Figure (2-8): Halides effect on the binding of prostate specific antigen of prostate cancer with ($^{125}$I-anti total PSA antibody). All other details are explained in the text.*

### 3.5.2.7. The Effect of Some Divalent Cations on the Binding of Prostate Specific Antigen of Prostate Cancer with($^{125}$I-Anti Total PSA Antibody)

Divalent cations such as $Zn^{++}$, $Mg^{++}$, $Ca^{++}$ were selected to investigate its effect on the binding of prostate specific antigen of prostate cancer tissue homogenate and $^{125}$I-anti total PSA antibody. Increased concentrations of these ions were selected as shown in figure(2-9). Magnesium and Calcium ions show a slight decrease in binding percent with raise of their concentrations while the most significant result in this experiment was in $Zn^{++}$ relative levels of binding. The curve in zinc ion was significantly enhanced at 10mm concentration to a very high binding percent 71.5%. Its known that zinc was considered as a regulator of PSA activity or as efficient noncompetitive inhibitor of PSA serine protease activity[149,150].

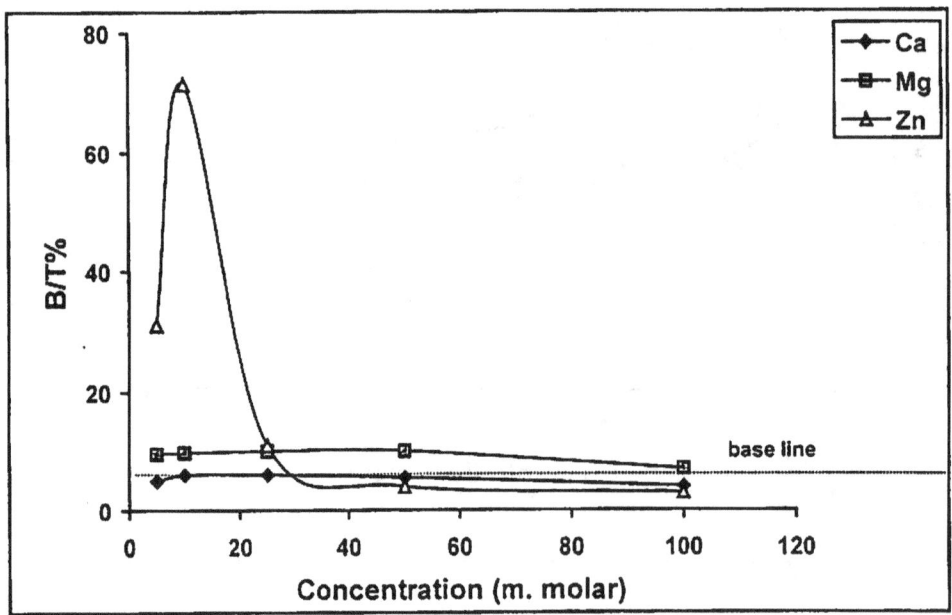

**Figure (2-9):** *Divalent cations effect on binding of prostate specific antigen of prostate cancer and ($^{125}$I-anti total PSA antibody). All other details are explained in the text.*

### 3.5.2.8. Polyethylene Glycol Effect on The Binding of Prostate Specific Antigen of Prostate Cancer with ($^{125}$I-Anti Total PSA Antibody).

The effect of high molecular weight polymer polyethylene glycol (PEG) was investigated. In figure (2-10) increased percent of polyethylene glycol was associated with a concomitant raise in binding percent with special focusing on 5% PEG concentration where there is a high alteration in binding percent value. The result was consistant with the speculation of Laurant[151] about the steric exclusion mechanism.

The total volume that contain the polymer and protein is fixed and equal to Vt. The volume that occupied by polymer and protein was represented by Vpo and Vpr respectively. Laurant assumed that.

Vt = Vpo + Vpr

Accordingly, any enhancement in the volume that occupy by the polymer Vpo by increasing the number or the size of the particle would reduce the volume that available for protein Vpr. Consequently that will increase the probability of collision and particle association to form the product.

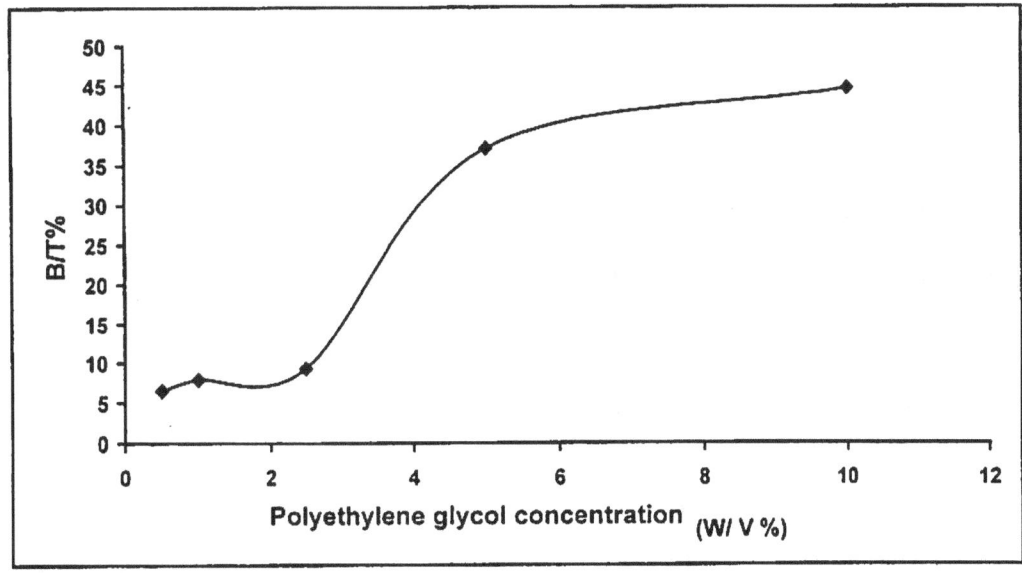

*Figure (2-10): Polyethylene glycol effect on the binding of prostate specific antigen of prostate cancer with ($^{125}$I anti total PSA antibody). All other details are explained in the text.*

## 3.6. The Kinetics Studies of the Reaction Between Prostate Specific Antigen of Prostate Cancer and ($^{125}$I-Anti Total PSA Antibody)

### 3.6.1. Determination of the Affinity Constant (Ka) and the maximal Binding Capacity of the Reaction Between ($^{125}$I-Anti Total PSA Antibody) and Prostate Specific Antigen of Prostate Cancer.

PSA and $^{125}$I-anti total PSA antibody reaction may represented by the simple reaction between antigen (Ag) and antibody (Ab) as in equation below.

$$Ag + Ab - I \underset{K_{-1}}{\overset{K_{+1}}{\rightleftharpoons}} Ag\,Ab - I$$

Where

$K_{+1}$ : Rate constant in forward direction.

$K_{-1}$ : Rate constant in backward direction.

Ag : PSA.

Ab-I: labeled antibody.

AgAb-I: the complex between PSA and its labeled antibody.

When the reaction at equilibrium point

$$Ka = \frac{K_{+1}}{K_{-1}} = \frac{[Ag\,Ab - I]}{[Ag][Ab - I]}$$

Where

Ka : equilibrium constant of association (affinity constant)

$$Kd = \frac{1}{Ka} = \frac{K_{-1}}{K_{+1}} = \frac{[Ag][Ab - I]}{[Ag\,Ab - I]}$$

Where

Kd : equilibrium constant of dissociation

Depending on the Scatchard equation which was discussed in section 2.11.1.

B/F= Ka (Bmax – B)

The values of the affinity constant(Ka) and maximal binding capacity were estimated. Figure (2-11) shows that Ka values were determined at four different temperatures 4,20,37,45$^0$C from the slopes of the straight lines that was constructed by using B/F values versus (B) values. Table (2-7) shows the values of Ka in ml.mg$^{-1}$. Its clear that there is elevation in Ka values with temperature consequently there was a shifting in equilibrium point to the direction of association (right) of the reactants with simultaneous decrease in Kd values.

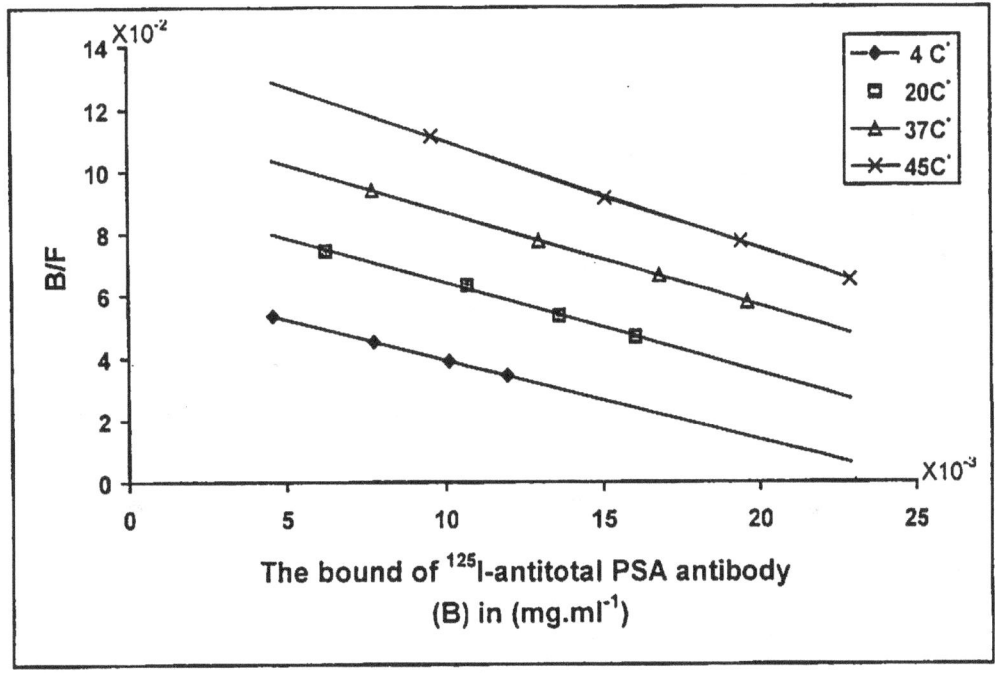

*Figure (2-11): Scatchard plot of the binding of prostate specific antigen of prostate cancer with ($^{125}$I-anti total PSA antibody). All other details are explained in the text.*

The straight lines that constructed in figure (2-11) by Scatchard plot reveals that the [125]I-anti total PSA antibody was directed against certain epitope and there was only one affinity toward it. This results indicate that prostate cancer tissue contains only one species of immunoreactive isoforms of prostate specific antigen and as mentioned by other investigators only free PSA is existed in prostatic tissue and there may be a negligible amount of PSA that bound to $\propto_1$-antichymotrypsin (PSA-ACT).

*Table(2-7): Equilibrium Constant of Association and Dissociation and Maximal Binding Capacity of The Reaction Between Prostate Specific Antigen of Prostate Cancer and ([125]I-Anti Total PSA Antibody).*

| Temperature $^0$C | Ka ml.mg$^{-1}$ | Kd mg.ml$^{-1}$ | Maximal Binding capacity mg.ml$^{-1}$ |
|---|---|---|---|
| 4 | 2.59 | 0.386 | 0.025 |
| 20 | 2.87 | 0.348 | 0.032 |
| 37 | 3.10 | 0.323 | 0.038 |
| 45 | 3.24 | 0.309 | 0.043 |

## 3.6.2. Determination of Kinetic Parameters of the Reaction Between Prostate Specific Antigen of Prostate Cancer and ([125]I-Anti Total PSA Antibody).

The time course of the reaction of PSA of prostate cancer tissue homogenate with [125]I-anti total PSA antibody was carried out to describe the kinetic parameters of the reaction. Figure (2-12) shows the time course of the formation of the complex ($^{125}$I-anti total PSA antibody: PSA) at four different temperatures.

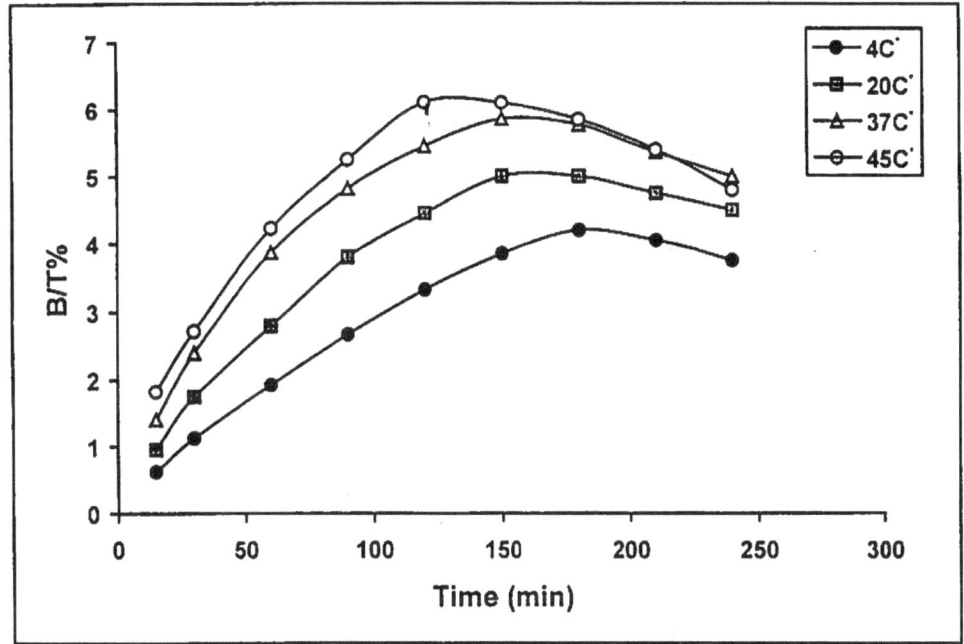

*Figure (2-12):Time course of binding of prostate specific antigen of prostate cancer with ($^{125}$I anti total PSA antibody). All other details are explained in the text.*

The biomolecularity of the reaction suggests that the reaction kinetic may achieve the following equation[152].

$$Ln(Ag\ Ab)e \left[ \frac{(Ab)T-(Ag\ Ab)_t\ (Ag\ Ab)e/(Ag)T}{(Ab)T\ [(Ag\ Ab)e - (Ag\ Ab)t]} \right] = K_{+1}.t. \left[ \frac{(Ab)T(Ag)T-(AgAb)e}{(Ag\ Ab)e} \right]$$

(Ab)T = Total antibody conc.(labeled anti body).

(Ag)T = total antigen conc.(PSA).

(Ag Ab)e = Concentration of the complex at equilibrium.

(Ag Ab)t = Concentration of the complex at time t.

But when the reaction obey the first order reaction kinetic the equation should simplified to be.

$$\text{Ln} \frac{(Ag\,Ab)e}{(Ag\,Ab)e - (Ag\,Ab)t} = K_{+1}.t. \left[ \frac{(Ab)T.(Ag)T}{(Ag\,Ab)e} \right]$$

However, only small amount of the ($^{125}$I-anti total PSA antibody) associated with the PSA to form the complex and the other part of the ($^{125}$I-anti total PSA antibody) was remained free in the reaction media. The binding percent was always low. This style of results was in general predominant through out our work therefore, the pseudo first order reaction kinetic conditions was available and the following equation was applicable.

$$\text{Ln} \frac{(Ag\,Ab)e}{(Ag\,Ab)e - (Ag\,Ab)t} = t.\,K_{obs}$$

(AgAb)e = complex conc. at equilibrium.

(AgAb)t = complex conc. at time t.

$K_{obs}$ = Observed value of first order rate constant

Figure (2-13) shows the $K_{obs}$ values at four different temperatures. $K_{obs}$ values was obtained from the slope of the straight line constructed using time of incubation versus $\text{Ln} \frac{(Ag\,Ab)e}{(Ag\,Ab)e-(Ag\,Ab)t}$ .The linearity indicated that the reaction obey the first order reaction Kinetic. $K_{+1}$ was determined from $K_{obs}$ values as follow:

$$K_{+}1 = K_{obs} \frac{(Ag\,Ab)e}{(Ag)T\,.\,(Ab)T}$$

Half-life time of complex association and dissociation was calculated with respect to the first order reaction kinetic rules

$$t_{1/2} = \frac{0.693}{\text{Rate constant}}$$

Table (2-8) contains the half–lives of association and dissociation at four different temperatures and the kinetic parameters.

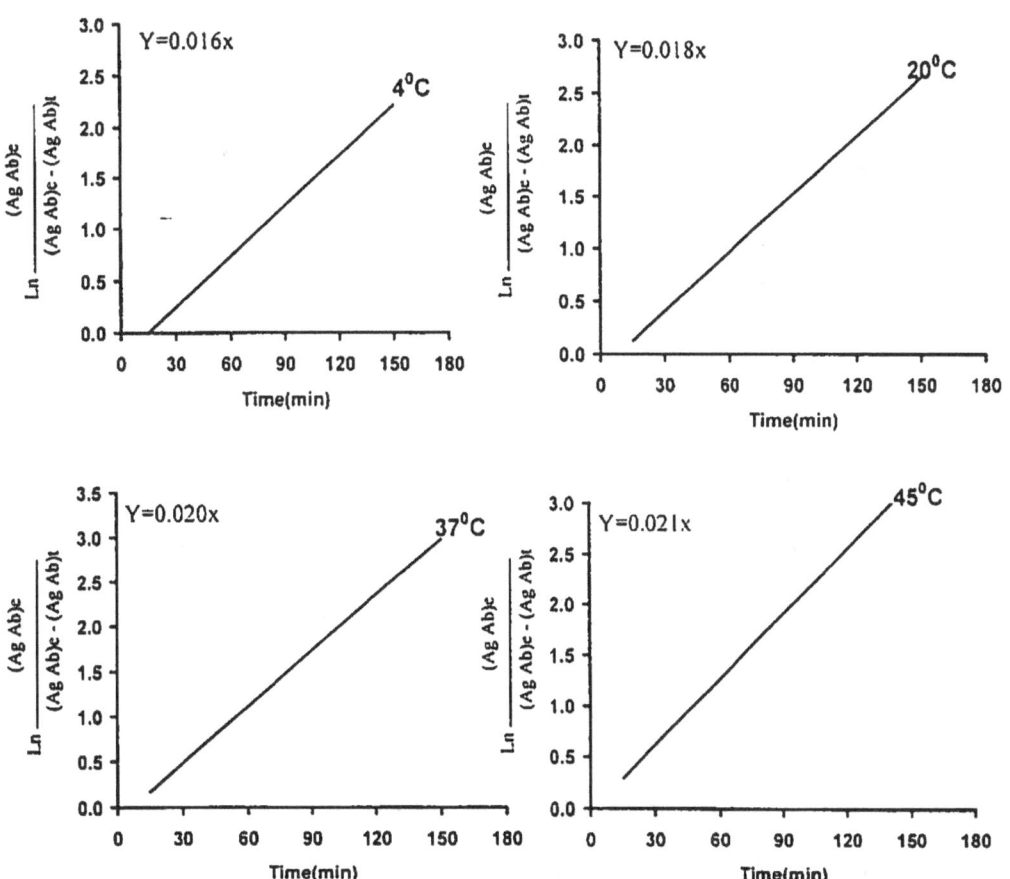

*Figure (2-13): Kinetic of the binding of prostate specific antigen of prostate cancer with ($^{125}I$ anti total PSA antibody). All other details are explained in the text.*

*Table (2-8): Kinetic Parameters of The Binding of Prostate Specific Antigen of Prostate Cancer with ($^{125}I$ Anti Total PSA Antibody).*

| Temp. $^0$C | $K_{obs}$ Min$^{-1}$.10$^{-3}$ | $K_{+1}$ ml.mg$^{-1}$.min$^{-1}$ | $K_{-1}$ min$^{-1}$ | $t_{1/2(ass)}$ min | $t_{1/2(diss)}$ min |
|---|---|---|---|---|---|
| 4 | 16.4 | 0.492 | 0.190 | 42.2 | 3.65 |
| 20 | 18.6 | 0.664 | 0.231 | 37.3 | 3.00 |
| 37 | 20.8 | 0.871 | 0.281 | 33.3 | 2.47 |
| 45 | 21.4 | 0.934 | 0.288 | 32.4 | 2.40 |

## 3.7. The Thermodynamics Study of the Reaction of Prostate Specific Antigen of Prostate Cancer and($^{125}I$ Anti Total PSA Antibody).

### 3.7.1. Thermodynamic Parameters of Standard State.

The reaction between prostate specific antigen of prostate cancer tissue homogenate and ($^{125}I$-anti total PSA antibody) was carried out with certain affinity constants which were shown in table (2-7). The dependence of affinity constants (equilibrium constants) on temperature can be observed through Vant Hoff plot as shown in figure (2-14). The results, which were obtained from Vant Hoff plot revealed that $\Delta H^0$ had low and positive value. The positive sign indicate that the reaction was endothermic and the low value of $\Delta H$ indicate that the favorable interaction between $^{125}I$-anti total PSA antibody and prostate specific antigen of prostate cancer tissue homogenate include only non-covalent interactions which are fundamentally electrostatic in nature such as charge-charge, dipole-charge, dipole-dipole, charge induced dipole, dipole-induced dipole interactions and hydrogen bonding.

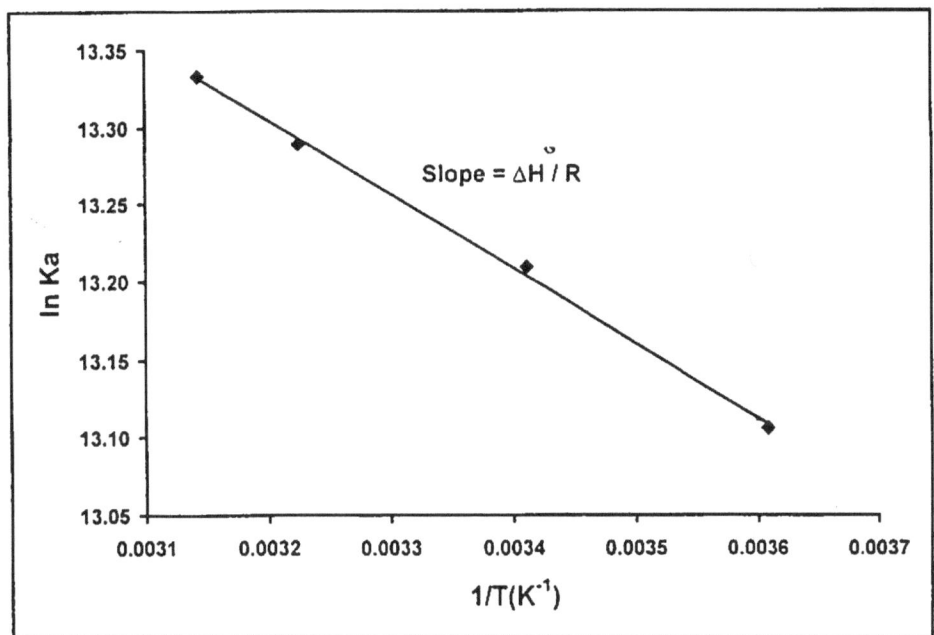

*Figure(2-14):Vant Hoff plot of the binding of prostate specific antigen of prostate cancer with ($^{125}I$ anti total PSA antibody). All other details are explained in the text.*

The sum of these types of interactions can yield some stabilization to the folded structure of the complex[153]. Table (2-9) shows the values of thermodynamic parameters of standard state at four different temperatures. The system is characterized by a high contribution of $\Delta S^0$ to the stability of the formed complex, while $\Delta H^0$ had a low effect. The high value of the positive $\Delta S^0$ suggested that the spontaneous binding was entropically driven[154].

*Table (2-9): Thermodynamic Parameters of Standard State Of ($^{125}I$ Anti Total PSA Antibody) Binding with Prostate Specific Antigen of Prostate Cancer Tissue.*

| Temperature °C | $\Delta H^0$ k.J. mol$^{-1}$ | $\Delta G^0$ k.J. mol$^{-1}$ | $\Delta S^0$ J. mol$^{-1}$. K$^{-1}$ |
|---|---|---|---|
| 4 | 3.96 | -30.201 | 123.27 |
| 20 | 3.96 | -32.195 | 123.35 |
| 37 | 3.96 | -34.261 | 123.28 |
| 45 | 3.96 | -35.269 | 123.31 |

## 3.7.2. Thermodynamic Parameters of Transition State:

The transition state theory proposed that the association of two reactants or more to form the final products is proceeds through the formation of an activated complex (transition state). Consequently, the interaction of $^{125}I$-anti total PSA antibody with PSA of prostate cancer tissue homogenate can be represented as follow:

$$PSA + Ab - I \longrightarrow [PSA \text{———} Ab - I] \longrightarrow PSA\text{-}Ab\text{-}I$$

Reactants             Transition State         Product

Ab-I = $^{125}I$-anti total PSA antibody.

The thermodynamic parameters of transition state($\Delta H^*$, $\Delta S^*$, $\Delta G^*$) could be determined from Arrhenius equation using kinetic constants. Figure (2-15) shows the Arrhenius plot of -ln $K_{+1}$ versus 1/T values. The slopes of the straight line represent the activation energy (Ea).

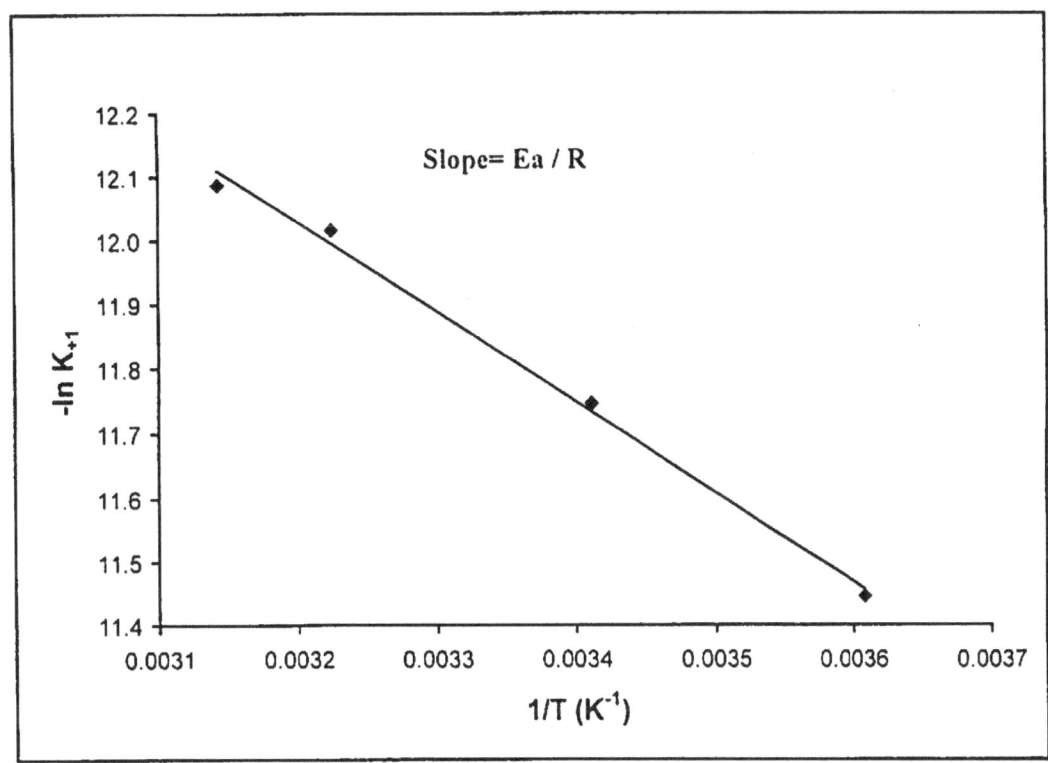

*Figure(2-15):Arrhenius plot of the binding of prostate specific antigen of prostate cancer with ($^{125}I$ anti total PSA antibody). All other details are explained in the text.*

Table (2-10) Shows the values of thermodynamic parameters of the transition state (Ea, $\Delta H^*$, $\Delta S^*$, $\Delta G^*$). Ea value represents the energy that required to overcome the energy barrier of the transition state for complex formation[155]. The value of activation energy was in accordance with the high positive value of $\Delta G^*$ which indicated that the formation of the activated complex is a non-spontaneous process. The high negative $\Delta S^*$ revealed that the activated complex had a more orderly structure than the reactants[156].

*Table (2-10): Thermodynamic Parameters of Transition State of the Reaction Between Prostate Specific Antigen of Prostate Cancer Tissue and ($^{125}I$ Anti Total PSA Antibody).*

| Temperature $^0C$ | Ea k.J. mol$^{-1}$ | $\Delta H^*$ k.J.mol$^{-1}$ | $\Delta S^*$ J. mol$^{-1}$K$^{-1}$ | $\Delta G^*$ k.J.mol$^{-1}$ |
|---|---|---|---|---|
| 4 | 11.67 | 9.37 | -115.1 | 41.27 |
| 20 | 11.67 | 9.23 | -115.3 | 43.05 |
| 37 | 11.67 | 9.10 | -115.7 | 45.00 |
| 45 | 11.67 | 9.03 | -116.3 | 46.04 |

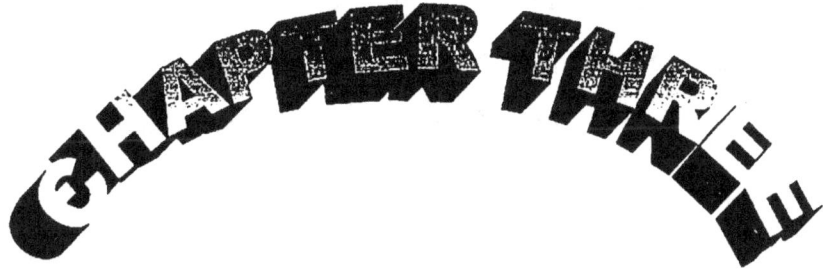

# SEPARATION AND CHARACTERIZATION
# OF
# FREE PROSTATE SPECIFIC ANTIGEN
# IN
# PROSTATE CANCER

## 1. Introduction:

Several studies have shown that the ratio of free to total PSA was lower in the circulation of prostate cancer patients than in BPH [29,157] Farther more, clinical studies have confirmed the efficiency of using this ratio to distinguish prostate cancer from BPH patients, particularly in the diagnostic gray zone at 4-10 ng. ml$^{-1}$ where the PSA concentrations overlap for cancer and non cancer diseases [158-161]. Also it has been suggested that the bound PSA as the major portion of total PSA would be a better discriminator between prostate cancer and benign prostatic hyperplasia than free PSA/ total PSA ratio, since bound PSA is apparently related to prostate cancer[162-165] and it could be candidate to enhance the discrimination power of PSA as tumor marker[166]. In contrast, other investigators reported that the determination of PSA-ACT and associated ratios do not improve the diagnostic impact to discriminate between prostate cancer and benign prostatic hyperplasia compared to free PSA/ total PSA ratio, but the ratios of PSA-ACT/ total PSA can be considered to be alternative tools of free PSA/ total PSA[167,168]. Recently, free PSA/ total PSA ratio mostly estimated by assays that use sandwich – type configurations based on the use of two monoclonal antibodies[169,170]. Monoclonal antibodies with specific characteristics as high sensitivity and specificity and equimolar binding to free PSA and PSA-ACT complex as well as the ability to distinguish between these two immunoreactive forms of PSA, have been reported by several authors[170-174]. Other investigators tend to use gel filtration chromatography to separate free PSA from PSA-ACT. They often use sephacryl S–300 or sephacryl S–200 as stationary phase with different flow rates to improve the performance of the gel[175,176].

# 2. Materials and Methods

## 2.1. Chemicals:

1-Sephadex. G-150 superfine from Phamacia Fine Chemical-Sweden.

2-Sepharose. CL-6B.

3-Gel filtration Calibration Kits from pharmacia fine Chemical-Sweden.

In addition to some other chemicals that mentioned in chapter two.

## 2.2. Apparatus

The same apparatus that used in chapter two.

## 2.3. Patients:

The patients with prostate cancer was divided to three groups with respect to tumor stages: stage B(7 patients), stage C(8 patients) and stage D(6 patients). The pooled sera of those groups were used latter in the experimental part.

## 2.4. Separation of Free ($^{125}$I-Anti Total PSA Antibody) from Complexed ($^{125}$I- Anti Total PSA Antibody) in Sera of Prostate Cancer Using Sepharose CL–6B.

### 2.4.1. Column Preparation:

The dimensions of the column were selected according to the following equations[177]

Column Length in (cm) = 30 × Column Diameter in (cm).

$$\text{Column Diameter in (cm)} = \left(\frac{\text{Protein Added in (mg)}}{10}\right)^{1/3}$$

Accordingly, the size of the column was ($1.1cm^2 \times 35.6cm$). The pre-swollen gel of sepharose Cl-6B was allowed to swell again with tris buffer pH7.4 then settled and excess buffer was decanted. The previous step repeated several times and the slurry gel was degassed and left for 24h at $4^0C$. The swollen gel was suspended and carefully poured into the column down the wall. After the gel had been settled, the column out let was opened. The addition of the gel was continued to reach the desired length.

A volume of 0.5 ml of blue dextron 2000 with concentration $2mg.ml^{-1}$ dissolved in tris buffer pH7.4 was applied to the column carefully, the flow rate was 12ml/hour.

### 2.4.2. Complex Separation.

1-A volume of 0.2ml of $^{125}I$-anti total PSA antibody was incubated at room temperature for 2hours with 0.2 ml of serum of prostate cancer patients.

2-Two tubes contained 0.2 ml of $^{125}I$-anti total PSA antibody was set aside for total radioactivity computation.

3-After incubation, the sample was applied to the surface of the column carefully.

4-The flow rate was adjusted to 12ml/hour and the fraction volume was 1ml.

5-The radioactivity of each tube was measured in addition to the total radioactivity by gamma counter.

6-Total protein content of each fraction was determined by lowery method[128].

*Calculations:*

1-The radioactivity of each fraction was plotted against the fraction number.

2-The area under peak was determined by the sum of the radioactivity in (CPM) of the fractions under peak.

3-The percent of complexed $^{125}$I-anti total PSA antibody to total $^{125}$I-anti total PSA anti body was calculated from the values of area under peak of each species

**2.4.3. Determination of the Molecular Weight of Free (125I-Anti Total PSA Antibody) and Complexed ($^{125}$I-Anti Total PSA Antibody) with Prostate Specific Antigen of Prostate Cancer.**

1-Sepharose CL–6B column that was mentioned in section (3.4.1) was calibrated by standard proteins (thyroglobulin 669kd, catalase 232kd), (ferritin 440kd, BSA 67kd) and (aldolase 158kd, ovalbumin 43kd) each couple of those proteins were dissolved in 1ml (according to the instruction of the manufacturers) of tris buffer pH7.4 and eluted together.

2-The flow rate was 12ml/ hour and the protein content of each fraction was measured by lowery method [128].

*Calculations:*

1-The partition coefficient $K_{av}$ of the eluted proteins were calculated using the following equation

$$K_{av} = \frac{V_e - V_o}{V_t - V_o}$$

Where

$K_{av}$:The fraction of the stationary gel volume which is available for diffusion of a given solute species.

$V_o$: Void volume.

$V_e$: Elution volume.

$V_t$: Total gel volume.

3-$K_{av}$ values were plotted versus log of molecular weight of the standard proteins.

## 2.5. Separation of Free Prostate Specific Antigen from Combined Prostate Specific Antigen in Sera of Prostate Cancer.

### 2.5.1. Column Preparations.

The dimensions of the column were selected according to the equations in section (3.4.1.) three gram of sephadex G–150 superfine was allowed to swell in excess of tris buffer pH7.4 (25ml of buffer per gram of gel) and left to stand for 72h at 4 $^0$c with out stirring to equilibrate with the buffer, then the buffer was decanted and the gel was resuspended in excess of buffer several times before packing in the column. Gel slurry was degassed and carefully mixed and poured into the vertical column that contains 5ml of the same eluent buffer. After the gel had settled the column out let was opened and more gel was added to reach the desired length. The column dimensions were (1.23 cm$^2$ × 37.5 cm). It was equilibrated with tris buffer pH7.4 for 24h. The void volume was determined as mentioned in section (2.4.1.) and the flow rate was 6ml/ hour.

### 2.5.2. Complex Separation.

1-A volume of 0.5ml of serum or tissue homogenate was applied to the surface of sephadex G–150gel filtration column. Elution was carried out using the tris buffer pH7.4. The collected fraction volume was 1ml for each fraction.

2-The total PSA concentration was measured in each fraction by immunoradiometric assay, which was mentioned in section (2.7.).

3-Total protein concentration in each fraction was measured by Lowry method that mentioned in section (2.6.).

## *Calculations:*

1-PSA concentration of each fraction was plotted against fraction number.

2-The area under peak was calculated as in section (2.4.2).

### 2.5.3. Determination of Molecular Weight of Free Prostate Specific Antigen and Combined Prostate Specific Antigen in Sera of Prostate Cancer.

1-Sephadex G–150 column that was mentioned in section (2.5.1) was calibrated by standard proteins (bluedextran 2000kd, BSA 67kd), (alkaline phosphatase 100kd, Chymotripsinogen25kd), (egg Albumin 43kd, ribonuclease 13.7kd) each couple of those standards were dissolved in 1ml (according to the instructions of the manufactures) of tris buffer pH7.4 and eluted together.

2-The flow rate was 6ml. hour and the protein content of each fraction was measured by lowery method [128].

## *Calculations:*

1-The partition coefficient $K_{av}$ was calculated as in section (3.4.3.).

2-The partition coefficient $K_{av}$ values were plotted versus log of molecular weight of the standard proteins.

3-Stock's radius of standard proteins were plotted against $(-logK_{av})^{1/2}$ to construct a linear calibration curve, then to determine the stock's radius of free PSA.

## 2.6. Most Appropriate Conditions of the Binding of Free Prostate Specific Antigen of Prostate Cancer with ($^{125}$I-Anti Total PSA Antibody).

### 2.6.1. The Effect of Different Concentrations of ($^{125}$I-Anti Total PSA Antibody) on the Binding with Free Prostate Specific Antigen in Prostate Cancer.

1-A volumes 6, 9, 12, 15, 18, 21, μl of $^{125}$I-anti total PSA antibody containing 27, 40.5, 54, 67.5, 81, 94.5 μg of protein respectively, where each was added to 100μl of free PSA solution (17.6 ng of PSA). The volume was made up to 300μl with tris buffer pH 7.4.

2-Other two tubes containing 21μl of $^{125}$I-anti total PSA antibody (94.5 μg proteins) where set aside for total radioactivity measurements.

3-All tubes were closed with parafilm tightly and incubated for 2h at room temperature with continuous shaking.

4-After incubation time, the tubes were centrifuged for 20min at 4$^0$C to precipitate the formed complex of (antigen–antibody).

5-The supernatant was decanted gentelly, and the pellet was washed with 200μl of tris buffer pH7.4, then the tubes were inverted on a filter paper for 10 min.

6-The rims of the tubes were swabbed with cotton and the radioactivity was counted by gamma counter.

## *Calculations:*

1-B/ T % was obtained as mentioned in section 2.10.1.

2-B/ T % was plotted against $^{125}$I-anti total PSA antibody concentration.

## 2.6.2. The Effect of Different Concentrations of Free Prostate Specific Antigen of Prostate Cancer on the Binding with ($^{125}$I-Anti Total PSA Antibody).

1-The volumes of 25, 50, 75, 100, 125, 150 μl of free prostate specific antigen containing 13.2, 26.4, 39.6, 52.8, 66, 79.2 ng of PSA respectively, was added to 12μl (54μg protein) of $^{125}$I-anti total PSA antibody.

2-The volume was completed to 300µl with tris buffer pH7.4 and two other tubes were contained only 12µl of $^{125}$I-anti total PSA antibody for total radioactivity measurements.

3-The tubes were incubated for 2hours at room temperature with continuos shaking.

4-After incubation time, the tubes were centrifuged for 20 min and the supernatant was disposed.

5-The radioactivity of the tubes were measured in addition to the total radioactivity.

## *Calculations:*

1-B/ T % was calculated as mentioned in section 2.10.1.

2-B/T% was plotted versus the concentration of free PSA of prostate cancer.

### 2.6.3. The Effect of pH on the Binding of ($^{125}$I-Anti Total PSA Antibody) with Free Prostate Specific Antigen of Prostate Cancer.

1-Different tris buffer pH 7, 7.2, 7.4, 7.6, 7.8, were prepared as mentioned in section 2.5.

2-A volume of 100µl (52.8ng of free PSA) of free prostate specific antigen was added to 12µl (54µg protein) of $^{125}$I-anti total PSA antibody. The total volume was made up to 300µl by one of the tris buffer that mentioned in step 1.

3-Two additional tubes contained 12µl of $^{125}$I-anti total PSA antibody were set a side for total radioactivity measurements.

4-After two hours of incubation, the tubes were centrifuged for 20 min and the supernatant were decanted.

5-The radioactivity of all the tubes was measured by gamma counter as well as the two tubes for total radioactivity determination.

*Calculations:*

1-B/ T % was calculated as mentioned in section 2.10.1.

2- B/ T % was plotted versus the corresponding pH value.

### 2.6.4. The Effect of Temperature on the Binding of Free Prostate Specific Antigen of Prostate Cancer with($^{125}$I-Anti Total PSA Antibody).

1-A volume of 12μl (54μg protein) of $^{125}$I-anti total PSA antibody was added to 100μl (52.8μg of PSA) of free prostate specific antigen of prostate cancer. The volume was made up to 300μl with tris buffer pH7.4.

2-The tubes were incubated for two hours with two additional tubes contained only 12μl of $^{125}$I-anti total PSA antibody for total radio–activity measurements.

3-The incubation was carried out at different temperatures 4,20,37, 45$^0$C

4-After two hours of incubation, the tubes were centrifuged for 20 min and the supernatants were decanted.

5-The radioactivity of all the tubes were measured including the tubes for total radioactivity computation by gamma counter.

*Calculations:*

1-B/ T % was calculated as mentioned in section 2.10.1.

2- B/ T % was plotted versus temperature degrees 4, 20, 37, and $45^0$C.

**2.6.5. Optimum Incubation Time for Binding of Free Prostate Specific Antigen Prostate Cancer with ($^{125}$I-Anti Total PSA Antibody).**

1-A volume of 12μl (54μg protein) of $^{125}$I-anti total PSA antibody was added to 100μl (52.8μg free PSA) of free prostate specific antigen of prostate cancer. The volume was made up to 300μl with tris buffer pH7.4.

2-Two additional tubes were contained with 12μl $^{125}$I-anti total PSA antibody and set aside for total radioactivity computation.

3-The tubes (except those for total radioactivity) were incubated for different periods of time 15, 30, 60, 90, 120, 150, 180, 210 and 240 min at $45^0$C.

4-After the incubation time of each tube. The tube was centrifuged and the supernatant was decanted.

5-The radioactivity of each tube was measured by gamma counter in addition to those for total radioactivity measurements.

*Calculations:*

1- B/ T % was calculated as mentioned in section 2.10.1.

2- B/ T % was plotted against the incubation time.

## 2.7. Kinetics Studies on the Reaction Between Free Prostate Specific Antigen of Prostate Cancer and ($^{125}$I-Anti Total PSA Antibody).

### 2.7.1. Determination of Affinity Constant and Maximal Binding Capacity of the Reaction Between the isolated Free Prostate Specific Antigen and (125I-Anti Total PSA Antibody).

1-A volume of 100μl (52.8μg of PSA) of free prostate specific antigen isolated from prostate cancer tissue was added to each of the volumes 3, 6, 9, 12, μl of $^{125}$I-anti total PSA antibody contained (13.5, 27, 40.5, 54μg protein) respectively.

2-The volumes were completed to 300μl with tris buffer pH7.4.

3-The tubes were incubated at $45^0$C for two hours.

4-The steps 1,2,3, were repeated at different temperatures 4, 20, 37°C.

5-After incubation time, the radioactivity of each tube was determined, then the tubes were centrifuged for 20 min and the supernatant was decanted.

6-The radioactivity of each tube was measured by gamma counter.

## *Calculations:*

1- B/ T % was calculated as mentioned in section 2.10.1.

2- B/ F ratio was calculated from B/ T value where F = T – B

F: the radioactivity, which represents the unbound part of $^{125}$I-anti total PSA antibody.

3-The concentration of the formed complex (B) was calculated as follow

$$B \ (mg.ml^{-1}) = \frac{B(cpm)}{T(cpm)} \ . \ \text{Tracer conc. in the incubation media (mg. } ml^{-1})$$

4-The affinity constant (Ka) and maximal binding capacity (B Max) where determined according to Scatchard equation.

$$\frac{B}{F} = Ka\,(B\,max - B)$$

5-Dissociation constant Kd was determined as follow.

$$Kd = \frac{1}{Ka}$$

6-The plot of B/ F versus B gave a linear relationship. The slope of the straight line represent Ka while the intercept of the straight line with (x) axis referred to B max value.

## 2.7.2. The Time Course of the Binding of Free Prostate Specific Antigen of Prostate Cancer with ($^{125}$I-Anti Total PSA Antibody).

1-A volume of 12μl (54μg protein) of $^{125}$I-anti total PSA antibody was added to 100μl (52.8μg of free PSA) of free prostate specific antigen of prostate cancer and the volume was completed to 300μl with tris buffer pH7.4.

2-Other two additional tubes contained only 12μl of $^{125}$I-anti total PSA antibody was set aside for total radioactivity computation.

3-The tubes were incubated at $45^{0}$C for different intervals of time 15, 30, 60, 90, 120, 150, 180, 210, 240, minutes.

4-The steps 1,2,3 were repeated with temperatures 4, 20, $37^{0}$C.

5-After incubation time the tubes were centrifuged and the supernatants were decanted.

6-The radioactivity of each tube was measured in addition to those two tubes for total radioactivity measurements.

## *Calculations:*

1- B/ T % was calculated as mentioned in section 2.10.1.

2- B/ T % was plotted against intervals of incubation.

## 2.8. Thermodynamic Studies on the Reaction Between Free Prostate Specific Antigen of Prostate Cancer and($^{125}$I-Anti Total PSA Antibody).

The practical part of the Thermodynamic Studies used the same equations that were mentioned earlier in section 2.12.

# 3. Results and Discussion

## 3.1. Separation of Free ($^{125}$I-Anti Total PSA Antibody) from Complexed ($^{125}$I-Anti Total PSA Antibody) in Sera of Prostate Cancer Using Sepharose CL-6 B.

Figure (3–1) shows the elution profile of the incubated solution which had contained sera of prostate cancer patients and $^{125}$I-anti total PSA antibody. Two peaks of radioactivity were appeared. The broad one or peak A represents the complex of $^{125}$I-anti total PSA antibody with different forms of PSA. Figure (3–2) shows some of these suggested complexes[178].

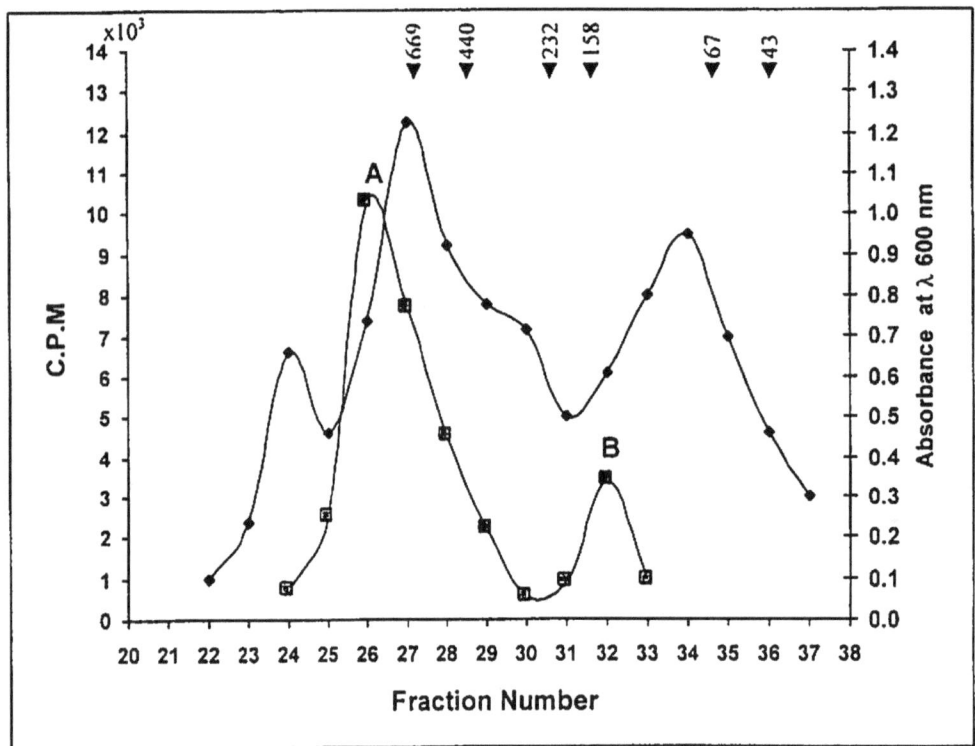

*Figure (3-1):The elution profile of the complex of ($^{125}$I-anti total PSA antibody) with isoforms of prostate specific antigen in sera of prostate cancer using sepharose CL-6B. All other details are explained in the text.*

Moreover, the high molecular weight of the first peak which was expected from its low retention volume may attributed to the PSA – [125]I- **anti total PSA antibody** polymerization and aggregation reaction which may indicate the bivalency or multivalency of PSA[179].

Also the idea of bivalency of PSA could be supported by the finding of Lilja *et al*[180], they found that the PSA – ACT complex (for example) covers three of the epitopes of PSA leaving at least two epitopes available to react with antibody, so that PSA may connected from both epitopes to produce a chain reaction and cause this enhancement in molecular weight.

The second peak (B) in figure (3-1) may represent the free [125]I-anti total PSA antibody. The high retention volume (32ml) indicate the presence of a relatively low molecular weight, approximately 150 kd. which was obtained from the calibration curve in figure (3–3).

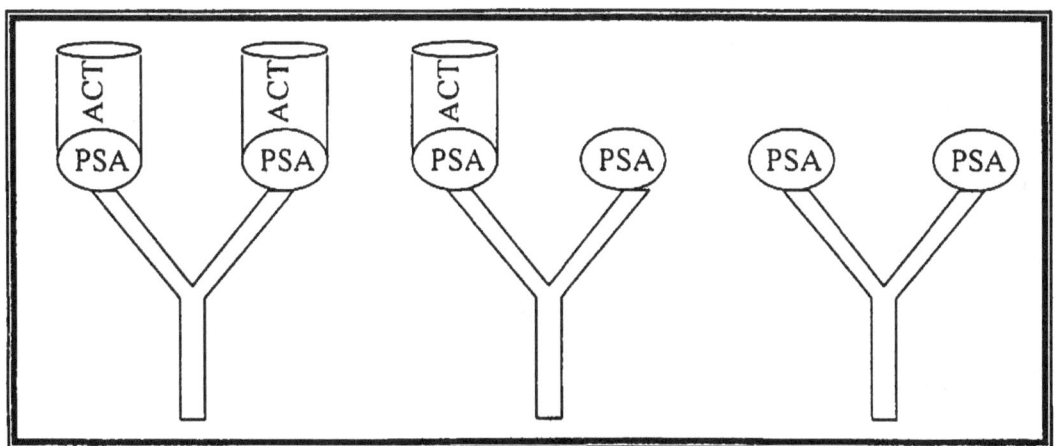

*Figure(3–2):The suggested complexes between serum prostate specific antigen and [125]I-anti total PSA antibody. All other details are explained in the text.*

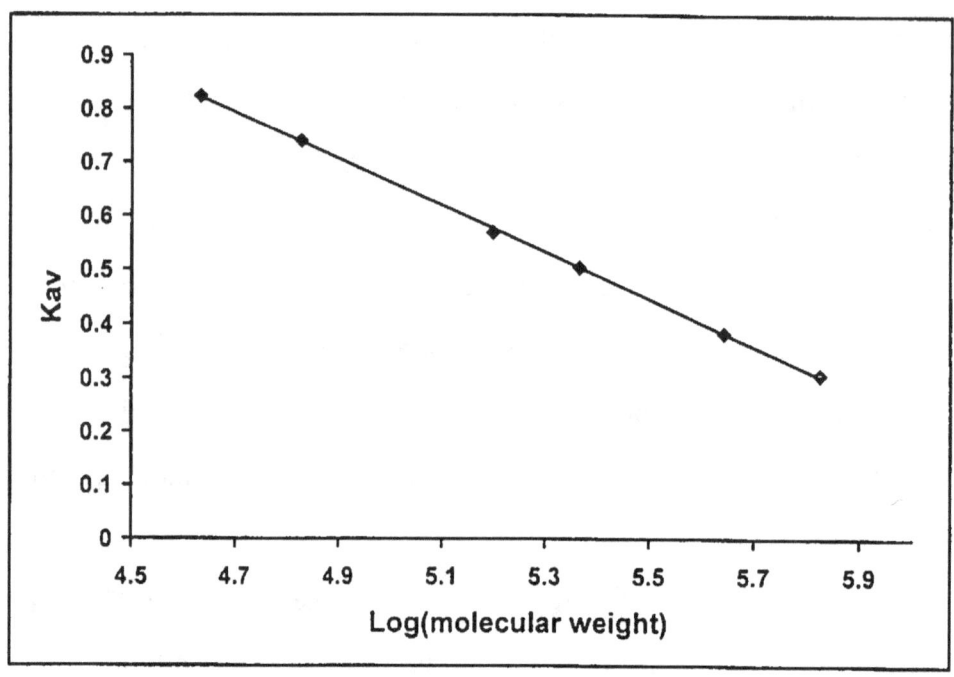

*Figure(3-3):Calibration curve for the determination of molecular weight of complexes of PSA isoforms with $^{125}$I-anti total PSA antibody by gel filteration chromatography using sepharos CL-6B. All other details are explained in the text.*

## 3.2. Separation of Free Prostate Specific Antigen from Combined Prostate Specific Antigen in Sera of Prostate Cancer.

Figure(3–4) displays two peaks A and B which represent, the two immunologically active isoforms of serum PSA the Combined PSA with $\alpha_1$-antichymotrypsin (PSA–ACT) and free PSA respectively. The chromatographic separation was performed depending on the significant differences in molecular weight between the two components. The molecular weights that obtained by the calibration of the gel column with standard proteins as shown in figure(3–5) was 32kd for free PSA and 96kd for the Combined PSA, in addition Stock's radius from figure(3–6) was obtained to be 25.8A˙ for free PSA and 44.75A˙ for the Combined PSA.

The obtained values of molecular weights were consistent with the values that were obtained by many other investigators[181-185].

In figure (3–4) the free PSA/ total PSA percent in sera of patients with prostate cancer stage B was 11.34%. This result was consistent with the value 11±7.2 % which was determined by Daniele *et al.*[186].

Other studies reported free PSA/ total PSA percent. It was 18% and up to 40% in cancer patients[187,188]. Most observations support the concept that there is a lower free to total ratio of PSA in prostate cancer patients if compared with patient with BPH[188]

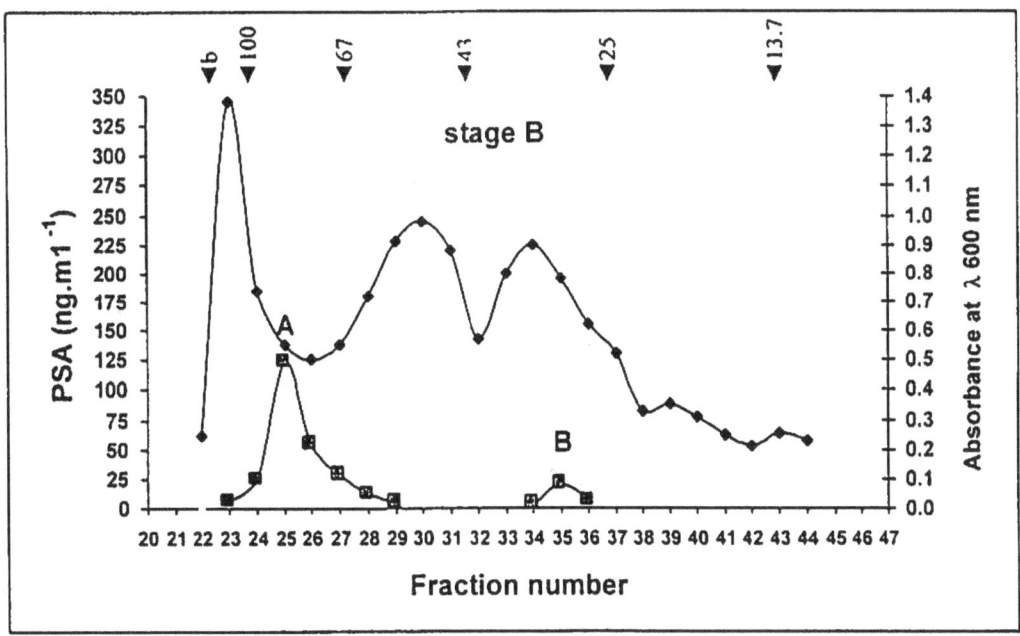

*Figure (3-4):Elution profile of prostate specific antigen in sera of patients affected by prostate cancer stage B using Sephadex G-150. All other details are explained in the text.*

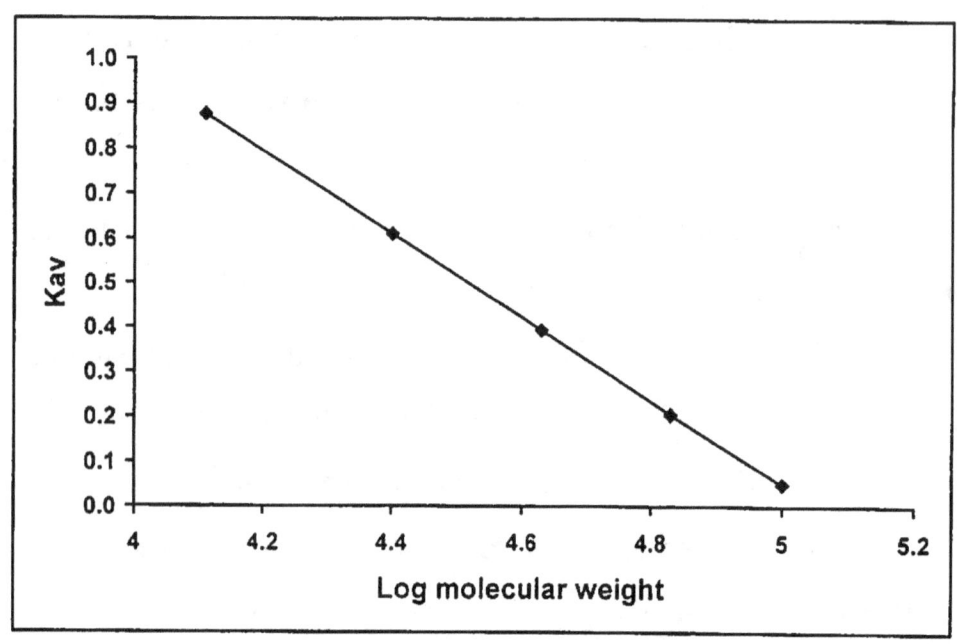

*Figure (3-5):Calibration curve for the determination of molecular weight by gel filtration chromatography using Sephadex G-150. All other details are explained in the text*

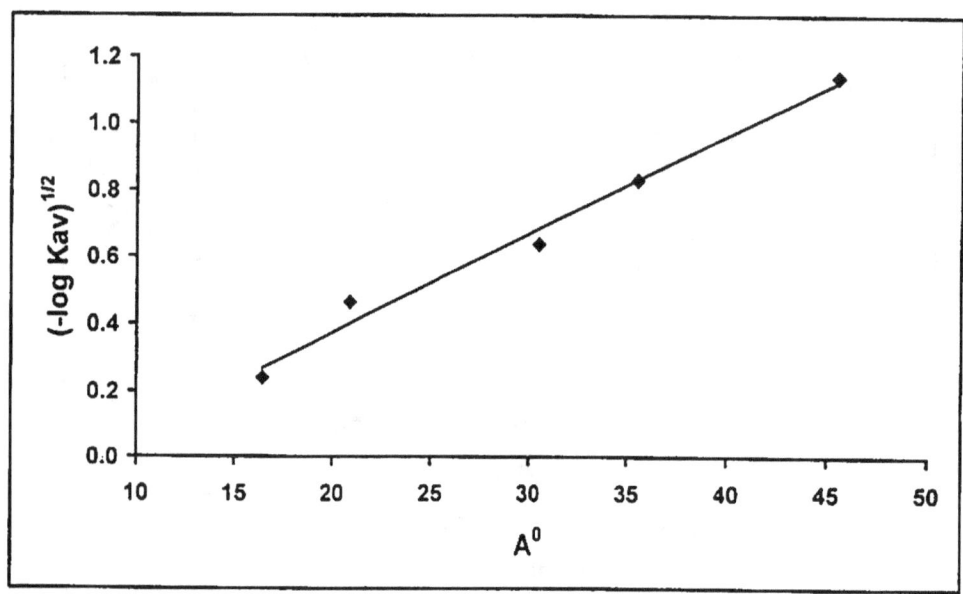

*Figure(3-6):Calibration curve for the determination of Stocks radius by gel filtration chromatography using Sephadex G-150. All other details are explained in the text*

In order to investigate the relationship between serum free PSA percent at different stages of prostate cancer, the serum of patient with prostate cancer of stage C and D were also eluted. Figure (3–7) displays the elution profile of pooled sera of patient with prostate cancer stage C. The peaks A and B, contain combined and free–PSA respectively and the percent of free to total PSA in stage C was 13.78 % as shown in figure(3-7).In figure(3–8) stage D displayed and the percent of free to total PSA was 13.5 % as it mentioned in table(3–1).

The results in table(3–1) which represent the free to total percent of PSA could not be used to differentiate well between local and metastatic cancer of prostate as locally confined and locally extended disease because there was no significant correlation between the obtained results of free to total percents of PSA at various stages of cancer. These results are in accordance with Charis *et al* [189] results, which show that the free to total PSA ratio is of no additional value in clinical staging of prostate carcinoma and the free to total PSA ratio is not a parameter of tumor load.

*Table (3–1): The Free to Total Prostate Specific Antigen Percent in Sera and Tissues of Prostate Cancer.*

| Sample | | No. | FPSA/ TPSA % |
|---|---|---|---|
| Serum of Prostate Cancer | Stage B | 7 | 11.34 |
| | Stage C | 8 | 13.78 |
| | Stage D | 6 | 13.5 |
| Tissue of Prostate Cancer | | 6 | 98 |

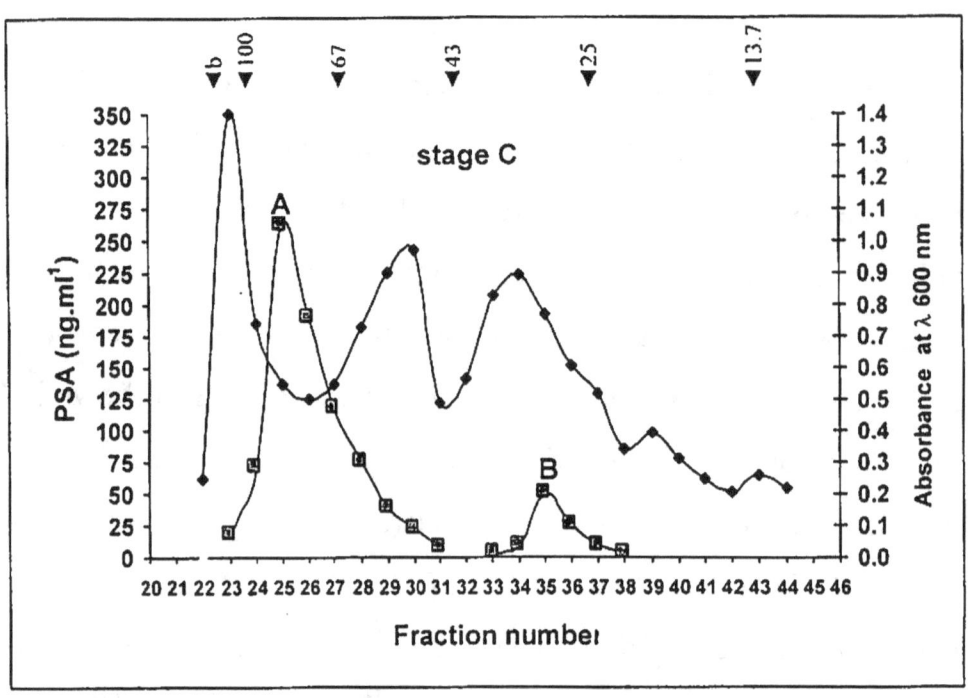

*Figure (3-7): Elution profile of prostate specific antigen in sera of patients affected by prostate cancer stage C using Sephadex G-150. All other details are explained in the text*

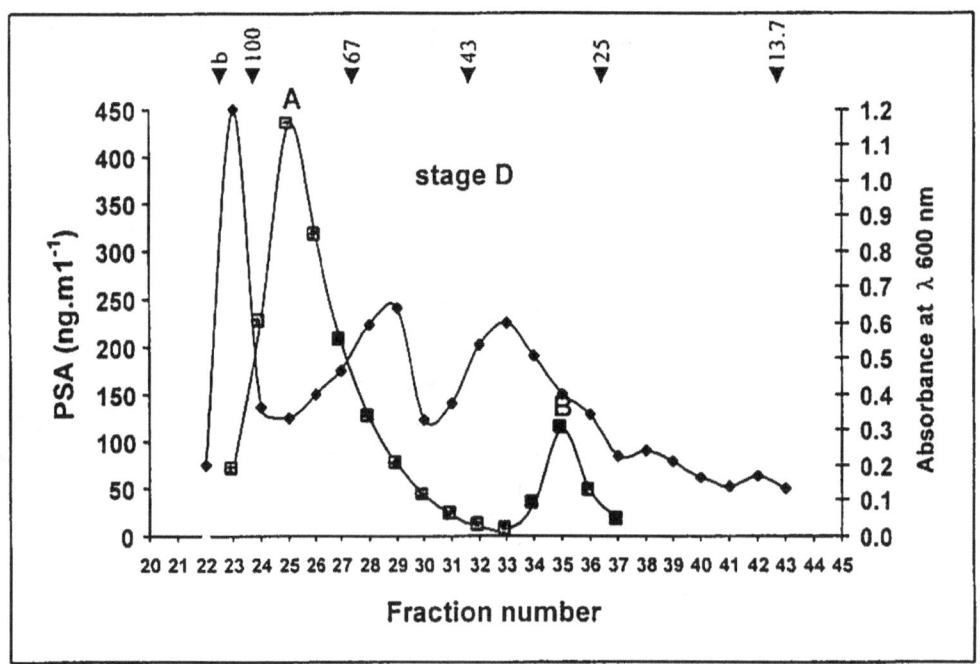

*Figure (3-8):Elution profile of prostate specific antigen in sera of patients affected by prostate cancer stage D using Sephadex G-150. All other details are explained in the text.*

Later, Jochen *et al*[190] mentioned that the free to total percents of serum PSA has been examined as a method to predict the final pathological stage of prostate cancer but, the relationship between this ratios and the stage of prostate cancer is controversial and the data could not confirm that f PSA/ t PSA ratio depend on tumor stage.

Figure (3-9) shows that the only immunologically active type of PSA in cancerous prostatic tissue is the free PSA. The absence of combined prostate specific antigen (PSA–ACT) in prostatic tissue homogenate is obscure. It had been speculated that the differences in PSA isoforms patterns between serum and tissue in prostate cancer are caused by additional complexes that occur in prostatic tissue[191].

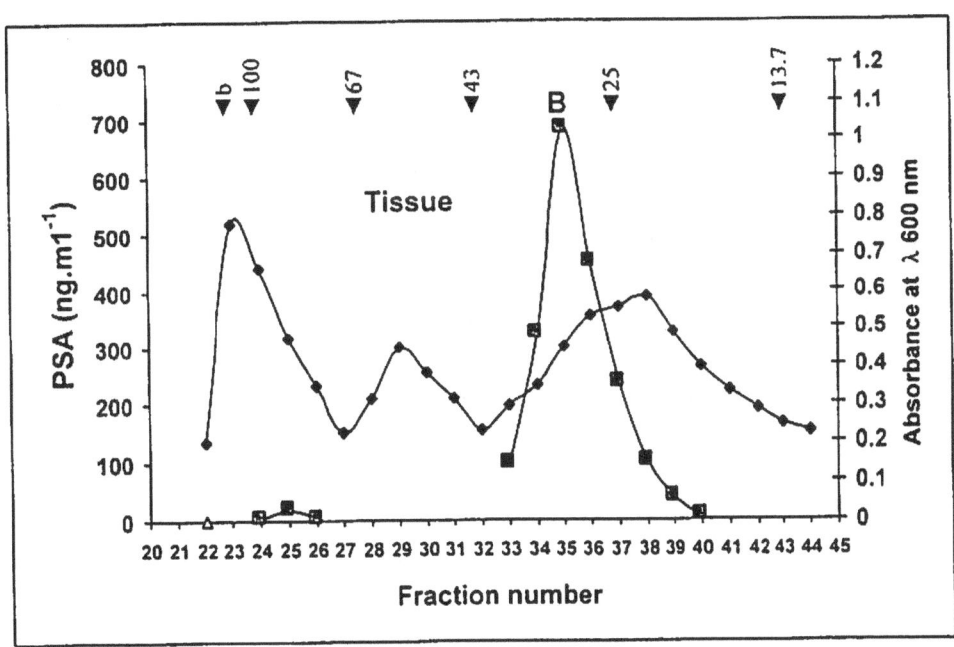

*Figure (3-9):Elution profile of prostate specific antigen in cancerous tissue homogenates of prostate using Sephadex G-150. All other details are explained in the text.*

Which prevent or reduce the formation of PSA–ACT[192,193]. This speculation was not consistent with our results because the association of PSA with other proteins in tissue to form a complexes must enhance the molecular weight of PSA, but in figure(3–9), the molecular weight of PSA was not enhanced and this putative speculation was doubtful.

In 1997, Yi *et al*[30] reported that zinc is a possible physiological inhibitor for the formation of PSA–ACT complex the physiological concentration of zinc in prostate is high enough to in activate or inhibit $\alpha_1$–antichymotrypsin and prevents the formation of PSA–ACT complex. With regard to the obtained molecular weight of PSA in prostate tissue. Yi *et al*[30] interpretations was acceptable and compatible with the results that obtained from figure(3–9).

However, the high concentration of zinc in prostate cancer tissue and the probability of the existence of other inhibitors was the suggested interpretations for the lack of PSA–ACT in prostate cancer tissue.

## 3.3. Most Appropriate Condition of the Binding of the isolated Free Prostate Specific Antigen from patients with Prostate Cancer and ($^{125}$I-Anti Total PSA Antibody).

### 3.3.1. The Effect of Different Concentrations of ($^{125}$I-Anti Total PSA Antibody) on the Binding with the isolated Free Prostate Specific Antigen from patients with Prostate Cancer.

Figure(3–10) display the effect of different concentrations of ($^{125}$I-anti total PSA antibody) on the binding with the isolated free PSA from sera of patients with prostate cancer. The optimum concentration of $^{125}$I-anti total PSA antibody was 0.18 mg. ml$^{-1}$

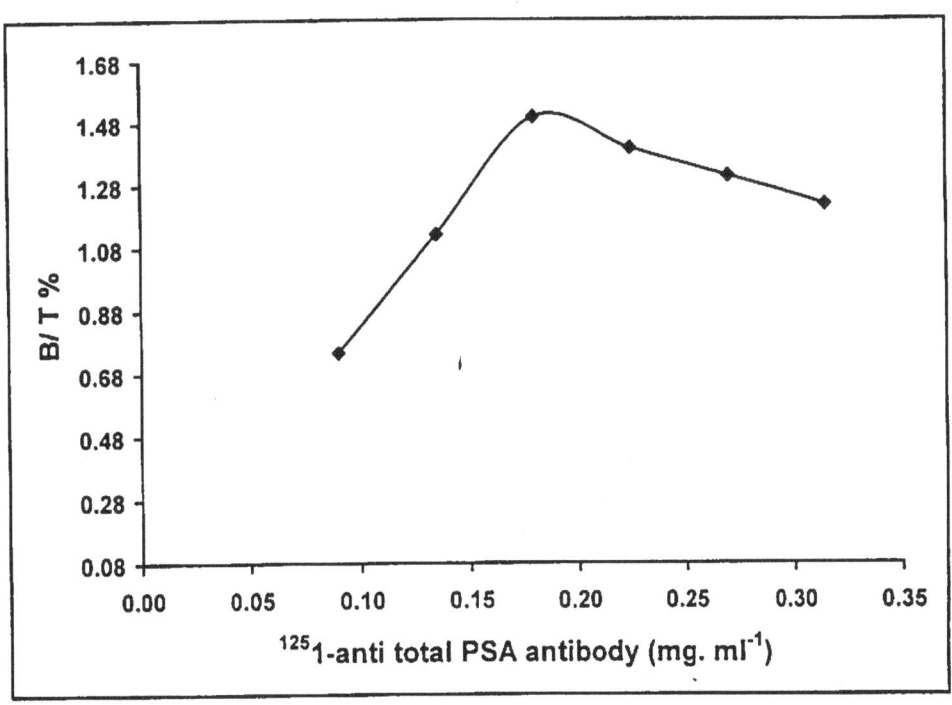

*Figure (3-10):The optimum concentration of $^{125}$I-anti total PSA antibody in the reaction with the isolated free prostate specific antigen from sera of patients with prostate cancer tissue. All other details are explained in the text.*

### 3.3.2. The Effect of Different Concentrations of the isolated Free Prostate Specific Antigen from sera of patients with Prostate Cancer on the Binding and ([125]I-Ant Total PSA Antibody)

Figure (3–11) shows the effect of different concentrations of the isolated free PSA from sera of patients with prostate cancer on the binding with [125]I-anti total PSA antibody. The optimum concentration was 176 ng.ml$^{-1}$.

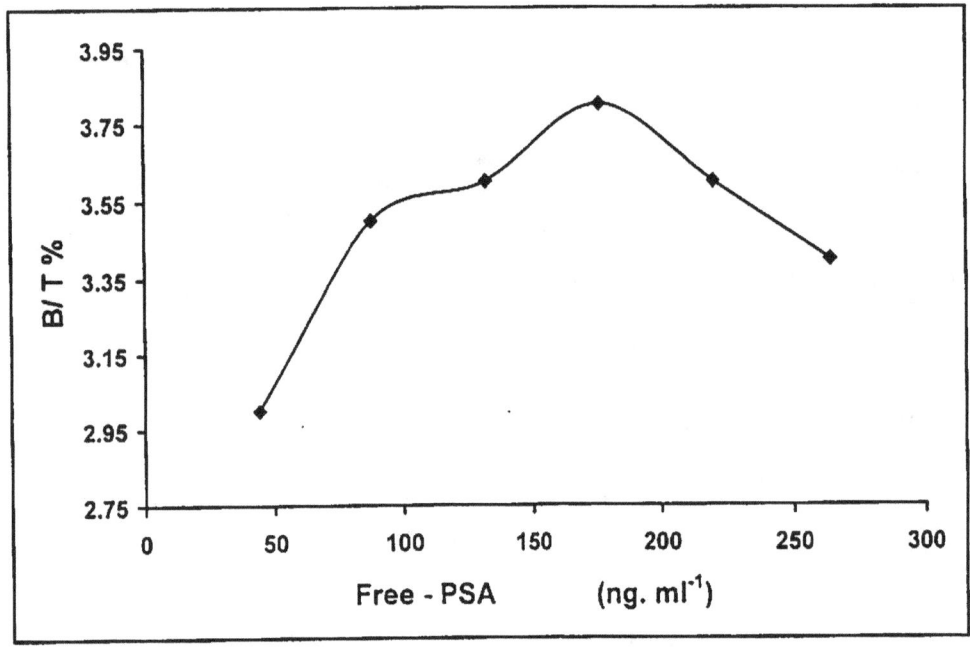

*Figure (3-11):The optimum concentration of the isolated free prostate specific antigen from sera of patients with prostate cancer in the reaction with [125]I-anti total PSA antibody. All other details are explained in the text.*

### 3.3.3. The Effect of Different pH on the Binding of the isolated Free Prostate Specific Antigen from sera of patients with Prostate Cancer and ([125]I-Anti Total PSA Antibody).

Figure (3–12) shows the optimum pH which produce a highest binding percent value through the reaction of free PSA that isolated from the sera of patients with prostate cancer and [125]I-anti total PSA antibody in different pH media. The optimum pH was 7.4.

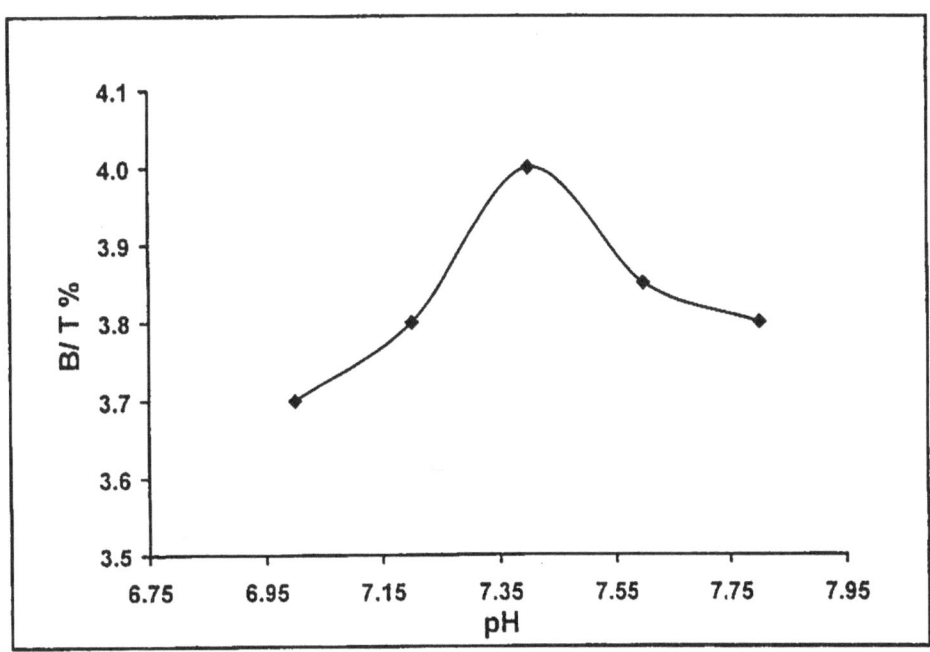

*Figure (3-12):The optimum pH for the binding of the isolated free-prostate specific antigen from sera of patients with prostate cancer and [125]I-anti total PSA antibody. All other details are explained in the text.*

### 3.3.4. The Effect of Temperature on the Binding of the isolated Free- Prostate Specific Antigen from sera of patients with f Prostate Cancer and ($^{125}$I-Anti total PSA Antibody).

Figure (3–13) shows the relationship between temperature and the binding percent between the isolated free PSA from sera of patients with prostate cancer and $^{125}$I-anti total PSA antibody. The most appropriate temperature for the binding was $45^0$C, therefore all next experiments were carried out at $45^0$C.

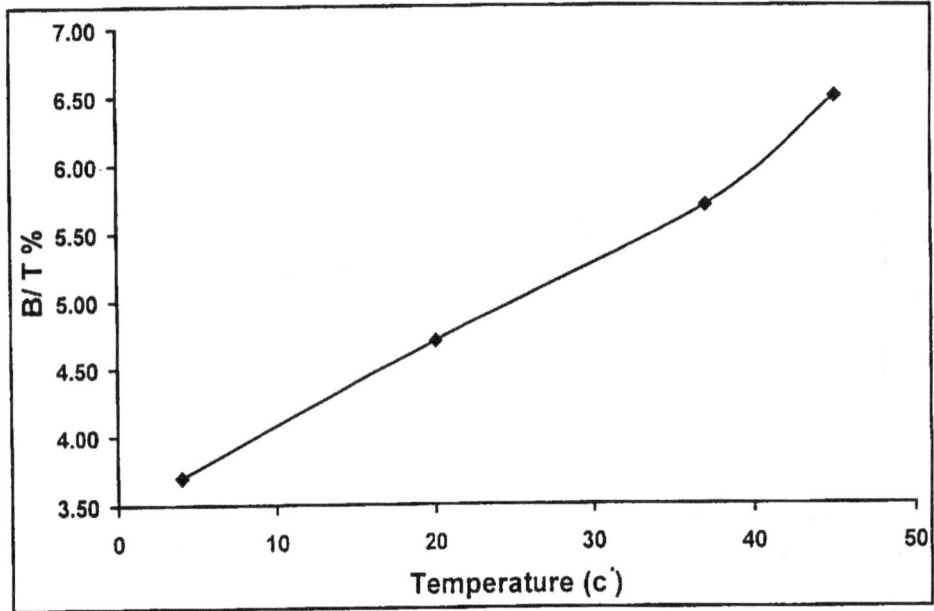

*Figure (3-13):The optimum temperature for the isoltated free prostate specific antigen from sera of patients with prostate cancer and ($^{125}$I-anti total PSA antibody). All other details are explained in the text*

### 3.3.5. The Most Appropriate Incubation Time for the Binding of the isolated Free-Prostate Specific Antigen from sera of patients with Prostate Cancer and ($^{125}$I-Anti Total PSA Antibody).

Figure (3-14) displays the optimum interval for the incubation of the isolated free PSA from sera of patients with prostate cancer and $^{125}$I-anti total PSA antibody. The highest binding between antigen and antibody take place after 120 min of incubation.

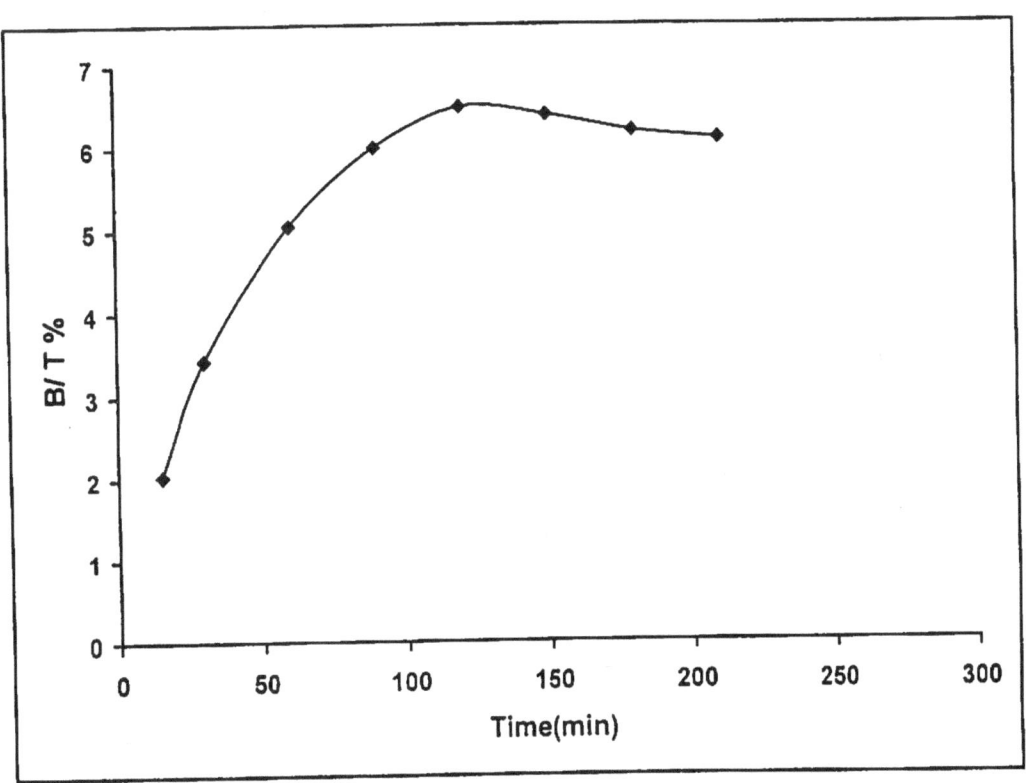

*Figure(3-14):Time course of the binding of the isolated free-prostate specific antigen from sera of patients with prostate cancer and $^{125}$I-anti total PSA antibody at $45^0C$. All other details are explained in the text.*

## 3.4. The Kinetic Studies of the Reaction Between the isolated Free-Prostate Specific Antigen from sera of patients with Prostate Cancer and ($^{125}$I-Anti Total PSA Antibody).

### 3.4.1. Determination of the Affinity Constant (Ka) and Maximal Binding Capacity (B max) of the Reaction Between (125I-Anti Total PSA Antibody) and the isolated Free-Prostate Specific Antigen from sera of patients with Prostate Cancer.

The reaction between free-prostate specific antigen which was isolated from the sera of patients with prostate cancer and $^{125}$I-anti total PSA antibody may be represented by the following equation:

$$fAg + Ab\text{-}I \quad \underset{K_{-1}}{\overset{K_{+1}}{\rightleftharpoons}} \quad fAg\,Ab\text{-}I$$

Where

fAg: free-PSA.

Ab-I: $^{125}$I-anti total PSA antibody.

$K_{+1}$: rate constant in forward direction.

$K_{-1}$: rate constant in backward direction.

At equilibrium.

$$Ka = \frac{K_{+1}}{K_{-1}} = \frac{[fAg\,Ab\text{-}I]}{[fAg][Ab\text{-}I]} = \frac{1}{Kd}$$

Where

Ka: Equilibrium constant of association (affinity constant)

Kd: Equilibrium constant of dissociation.

Figure (3-15) represents the application of Scatchard equation.

$$\frac{B}{F} = Ka\,(B\,max\text{-}B)\ \text{as mentioned in section 2.7.1.}$$

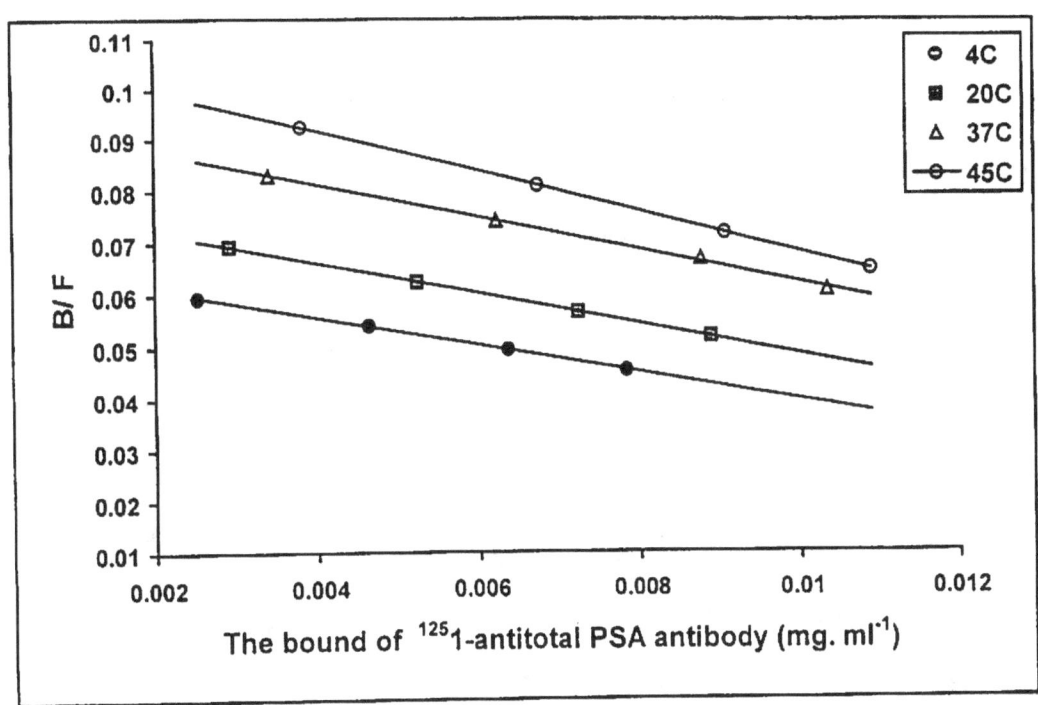

*Figure (3-15): Scatchard plot of the binding of the isolated free-prostate specific antigen from sera of patients with prostate cancer and $^{125}I$-anti total PSA antibody. All other details are explained in the text.*

The affinity constants Ka and maximal binding capacities were determined at four different temperatures 4, 20, 37, 45 C

Table (3-2) contains these results and the values of the equilibrium constants of dissociation.

The necessary step in the kinetic study of free PSA was the isolation of free PSA from combined PSA. The used antibody or $^{125}$I-anti total PSA antibody had the ability to recognize the specific epitopes that present on the surface of both free PSA and PSA-ACT, and because of the relatively small size of (approximately 30kd) free-PSA, it may has the potential to react with [125]I-anti total PSA antibody faster than PSA-ACT (approximately 100kd)[30]. The reaction with two different isoforms of PSA results in two different affinity constants and a curvature in the straight lines of Scatchard plot. The interference of Ka values in the same plot may hinder the estimation of Ka value of free PSA.

*Table (3-2): Equilibrium Constants and Maximal Binding Capacity of the Reaction Between the isolated Free-Prostate Specific Antigen from sera of patients with Prostate Cancer and ([125]I-Anti Total PSA Antibody).*

| Temperature C° | Ka ml. mg$^{-1}$ | Kd mg. ml$^{-1}$ | Maximal Binding capacity mg. ml$^{-1}$ |
|:---:|:---:|:---:|:---:|
| 4 | 2.67 | 0.375 | 0.025 |
| 20 | 2.97 | 0.337 | 0.026 |
| 37 | 3.24 | 0.309 | 0.029 |
| 45 | 3.38 | 0.296 | 0.031 |

The values of Ka and Kd of the isolated free-PSA from sera of patients with prostate cancer were comparable with those of tissues of prostate cancer patients in table(2-7). The similarity in the equilibrium constants of the two reactions with temperature change may reflect that the two species were very close together in structure.

## 3.4.2. Determination of Kinetic Parameters of the Reaction Between the isolated Free-Prostate Specific Antigen from sera of patients with Prostate Cancer and ($^{125}$I-Anti Total PSA Antibody).

The time course of $^{125}$I-anti total PSA antibody binding with isolated free PSA from sera of patients with prostate cancer was carried out to describe kinetic parameters of the reaction. Figure (3-16) show the time course of complex formation at four different temperatures.

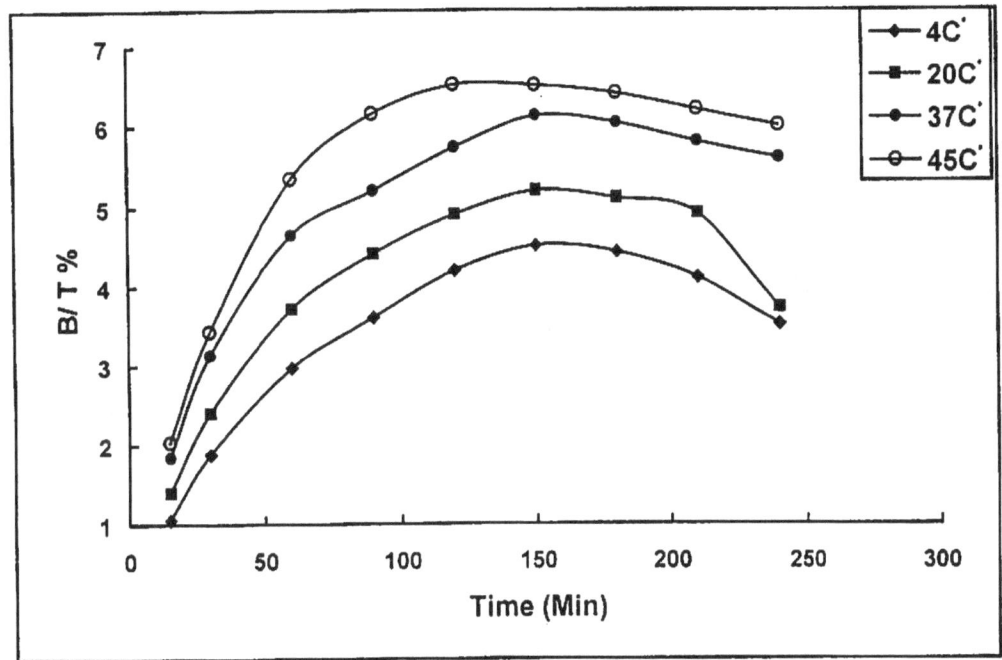

*Figure (3-16): Time course of the binding of the isolated free-prostate specific antigen from sera of patients with prostate cancer and $^{125}$I-anti total PSA antibody. All other details are explained in the text.*

The data of time course was consistent with first order reaction kinetics so that the following equation was applicable.

$$\ln \frac{(fAg\ Ab)e}{(fAg\ Ab)e-(fAg\ Ab)t} = t.\ Kobs.$$

(fAg Ab)e: concentration of the complex at equilibrium.

(fAg Ab)t: concentration of the complex at time t.

$K_{obs}$: The observed value of first order reaction Kinetic.

$K_{obs}$ values were estimated at four different temperature points in figure

(3-17) depending on the linear relationship between time t and ln[(fAg Ab)e/(fAg Ab)e-(fAg Ab)t], where the slope of the straight line represents the $K_{obs}$ value.

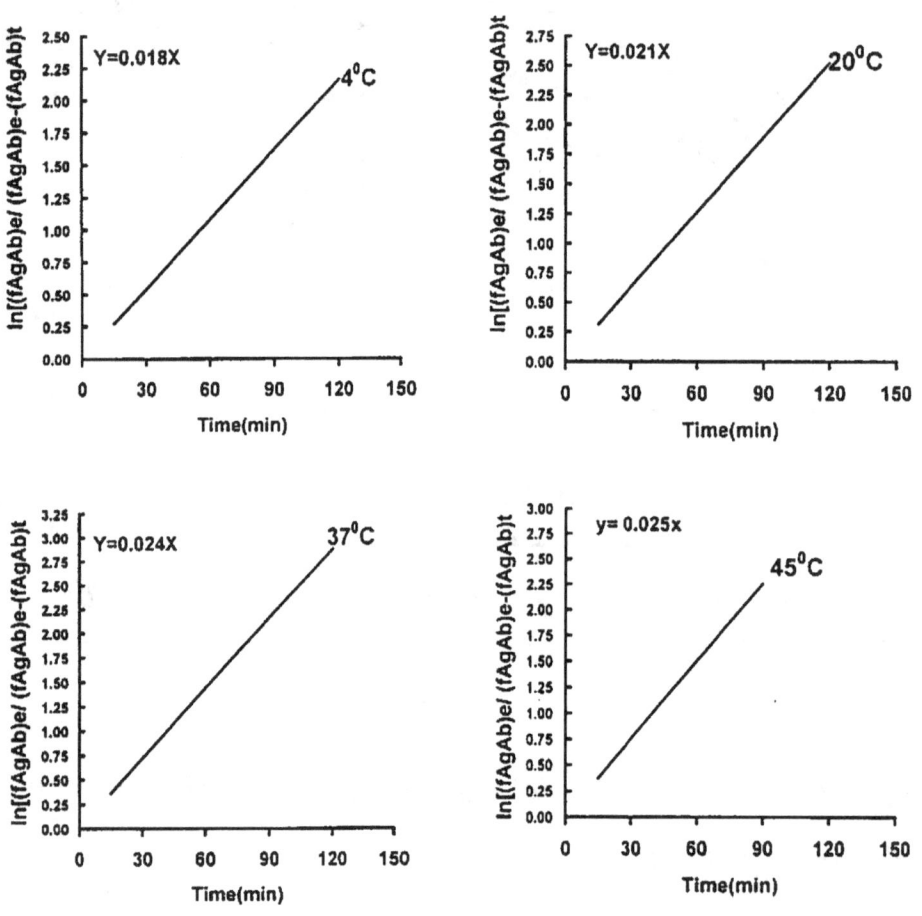

*Figure (3-17): Kinetic of binding of the isolated free-prostate specific antigen from sera of patients with prostate cancer with $^{125}$I-anti total PSA antibody. All other details are explained in the text.*

Other Kinetic parameters were calculated as mentioned in section 3.6.2.

Table (3-3) show those parameters in detail. The $K_{+1}$ values were little higher than those of PSA of prostate tissue in table (2-8) which indicates that the reaction of the isolated free PSA from sera was faster than the reaction of PSA of prostatic tissue using the same antibody. The differences in $K_{+1}$ values may be attributed to the difference in the contents of the reaction media[194].

*Table (3-3): Kinetic Parameters of the Binding of the isolated Free-Prostate Specific Antigen from sera of patients with Prostate Cancer and ($^{125}I$-Anti Total PSA Antibody) at Different Temperatures.*

| Temperature $^0C$ | $K_{obs}$ min$^{-1}$ | $K_{+1}$ ml. mg$^{-1}$. min$^{-1}$ | $K_{-1}$ min$^{-1}$ | $t_{1/2 \text{ (ass)}}$ min | $t_{1/2(diss)}$ min |
|---|---|---|---|---|---|
| 4 | 0.018 | 4.6 | 0.217 | 38.5 | 3.194 |
| 20 | 0.021 | 6.2 | 0.161 | 33.0 | 4.31 |
| 37 | 0.024 | 8.3 | 0.120 | 28.9 | 5.78 |
| 45 | 0.025 | 9.7 | 0.109 | 27.7 | 6.36 |

## 3.5 Thermodynamic Study of Reaction Between the isolated Free Prostate Specific Antigen from sera of patients with Prostate Cancer and ($^{125}$I-Anti Total PSA Antibody).

### 3.5.1. Thermodynamic Parameters of Standard State.

The relationship between the equilibrium constant (affinity constant) and temperature of the reaction between $^{125}$I-anti total PSA antibody and the isolated free PSA from sera of patients with prostate cancer could be observed through Vant Hoff plot in figure (3-18).

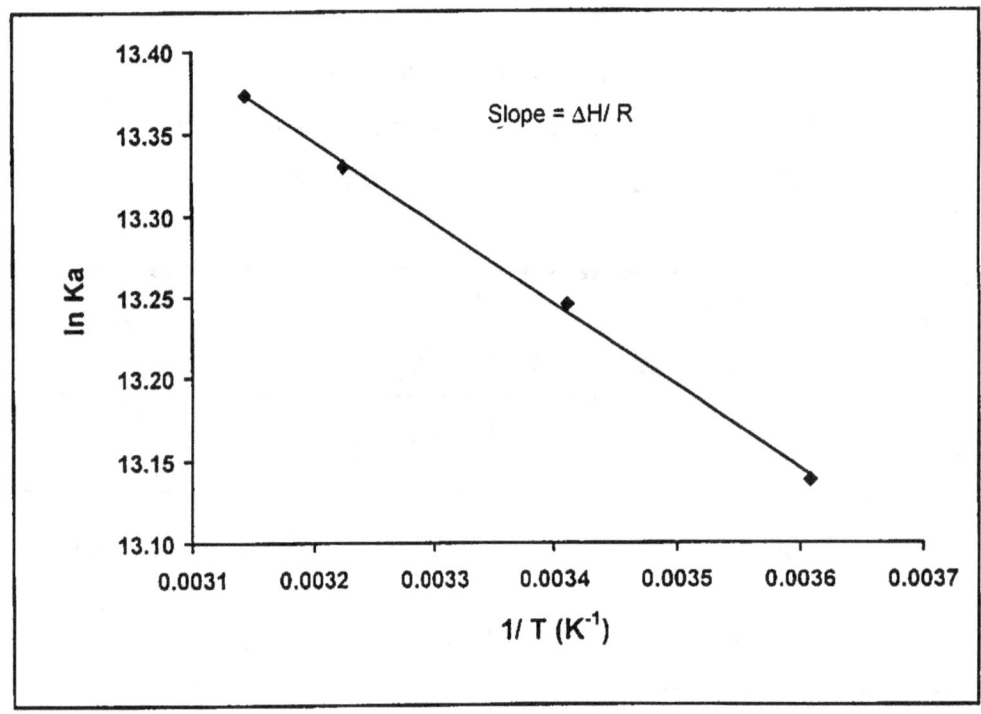

*Figure (3-18): Vant Hoff plot of the reaction between the isolated free prostate specific antigen from sera of patients with prostate cancer and ($^{125}$I- Anti Total PSA Antibody). All other details are explained in the text.*

The $\Delta H^0$ was obtained from the slope of Vant Hoff plot and the positive sign of $\Delta H^0$ indicate that the reaction is endothermic. Other thermodynamic parameters are reported in table (3-4). The relatively low values of $\Delta H^0$ may shed a light on the nature of the interaction between the reactants. Within the calculated $\Delta H^0$ values the favorable interaction was non-covalent interaction such as (charge-charge), (charge-dipole), (dipole-dipole), (charge-induced dipole), (dipole- induced dipole) in addition to hydrogen bonds[153].

*Table (3-4): Thermodynamic Parameters of Standard State of the Reaction Between the isolated Free-Prostate Specific Antigen from sera of Patients with Prostate Cancer and ($^{125}$I-Anti Total PSA Antigen).*

| Temperature C | $\Delta H^0$ k. J. mol$^{-1}$ | $\Delta G^0$ k. J. mol$^{-1}$ | $\Delta s^0$ J. mol$^{-1}$. K$^{-1}$ |
|---|---|---|---|
| 4 | 4.203 | -30.274 | 124.4 |
| 20 | 4.203 | -32.282 | 124.4 |
| 37 | 4.203 | -34.374 | 124.4 |
| 45 | 4.203 | -35.374 | 124.4 |

The negative sign of $\Delta G^0$ values in table (3-4) revealed that the formed complex was highly stable. Our system is characterized by a high contribution of $\Delta S^0$ and to less extent $\Delta H^0$ in the stability of the formed complex[148].

The results in table (3-4) are comparable with those obtained in table (2-9) resulted from the reaction of $^{125}$I-anti total PSA antibody with PSA of prostate cancer tissue homogenate. The result's comparability may reflect that the structure of free-PSA in sera of prostate cancer is very close or identical with that of the PSA in prostatic tissue.

### 3.5.2. The Thermodynamic Parameters of Transition State.

The thermodynamic parameters of transition state of the reaction between the isolated free PSA from sera of patients with prostate cancer and $^{125}$I-anti total PSA antibody were obtained from Arrhenius plot. The slope of the straight line in figure (2-16) represents the activation energy (Ea).

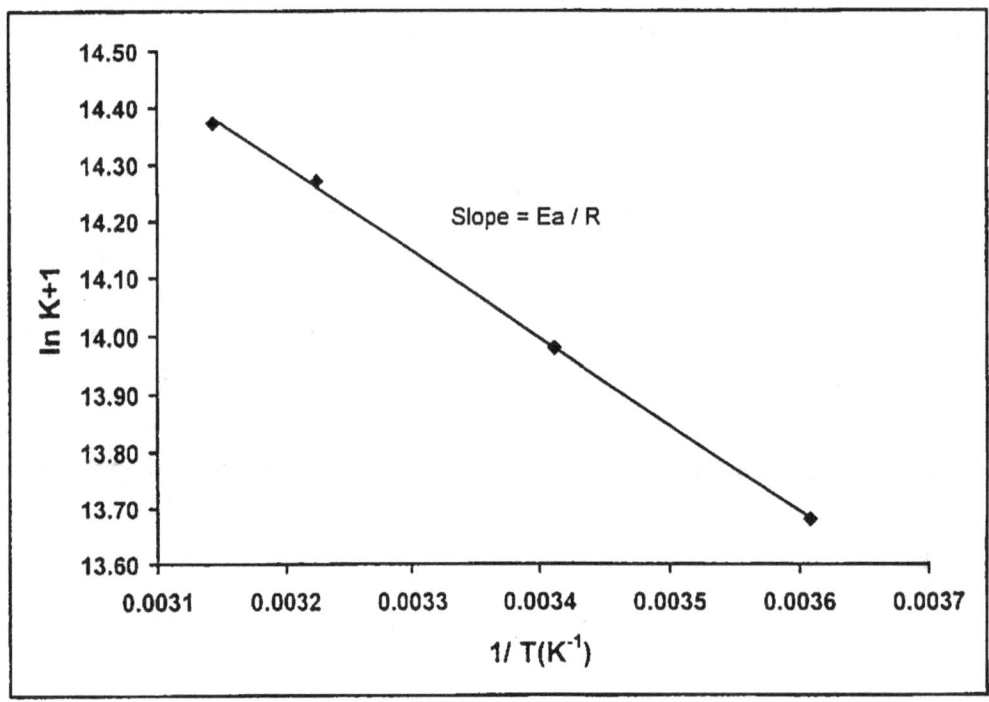

*Figure(2-16):Arrhenius plot of the binding of the isolated free-prostate specific antigen from sera of patients with prostate cancer with ($^{125}$I-anti total PSA antibody). All other details are explained in the text.*

The high activation energy value ($12.38 \text{k.J.mol}^{-1}$) is in accordance with the high positive values of $\Delta G^*$ which indicate that the formation of the activated complex is non-spontaneous process and required a lot of energy to over come the transition state energy barrier[155].

Other parameters of transition state are shown in table (3-5).

*Table (3-5): Thermodynamic Parameters of Transition State of the Reaction between the isolated Free-Prostate Specific Antigen from Sera of Patients with Prostate Cancer and ($^{125}$I-Anti Total PSA Antibody).*

| Temperature $^0C$ | Ea k. J. mol$^{-1}$ | $\Delta H^*$ k. J. mol$^{-1}$ | $\Delta G^*$ k. J. mol$^{-1}$ | $\Delta S^*$ J. mol$^{-1}$. K$^{-1}$ |
|---|---|---|---|---|
| 4 | 12.38 | 10.076 | 36.187 | -94 |
| 20 | 12.38 | 9.943 | 37.686 | -94 |
| 37 | 12.38 | 9.802 | 39.264 | -94 |
| 45 | 12.38 | 9.735 | 40.075 | -95 |

The high negative sign of $\Delta S^*$ reveals that the activated complex had a more orderly structure than the reactants[156].

However, the thermodynamic data indicated that the binding between the isolated free PSA from sera of patients with prostate cancer and $^{125}$I-anti total PSA antibody was mainly entropically driven.

The mean value of $\Delta G^*$ of the reaction between $^{125}$I-anti total PSA antibody and PSA of prostate cancer tissue homogenate in table (2-10) is approximately $44 \text{k.J.mol}^{-1}$ while that of the isolated free PSA from sera of patients with prostate cancer was $38k.J.mol^{-1}$. The differences in $\Delta G^*$ values indicate that there are differences in the stability of the two formed complexes which may be attributed to the differences in media contents.[194]

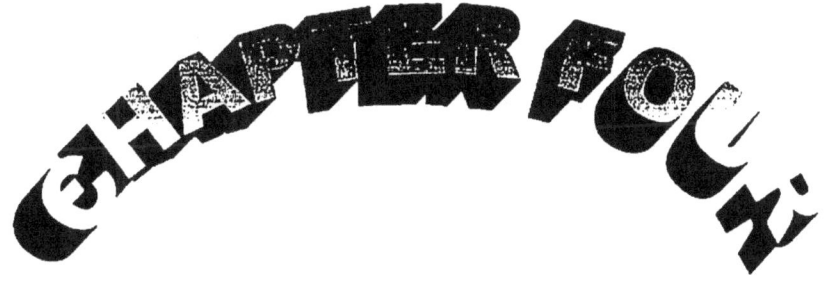

# EVALUATION OF THE ROLE
# OF
# ZINC IN SERA AND TISSUES
# OF
# PATIENTS WITH PROSTATE CANCER

# 1. Introduction:

Zinc (Zn) is an essential nutrient for many plants[195], animals[196] and microorganisms[197]. The essentiality of zinc for human was first demonstrated when arrested sexual development in adolescent children was reversed with zinc supplements[198]. Zinc is the second most abundant trace metal found in eukaryotic organism, second only to iron if one subtracted the amount of iron found in hemoglobin, zinc become the most abundant trace element found in human body[199]. Normal human body contains (2-3) gm of zinc in adulthood. Many sites in human body like muscle, liver, pancreas, skin and bone comprise most of body zinc reserve, nevertheless the heavy metal is more a abundant in human prostate gland than in other organs[200]. The biochemical basis for the essentiality of zinc is not completely understood. Although it is an essential cofactor for more than 200 metalloenzymes[201]. In blood normal levels of zinc was estimated in serum nutrophile, lymphocyte and erythrocyte by using the flame atomic absorption spectrophotometer. The data which was obtained by this method indicate that the 75-88% of total zinc content of normal human blood is contained in red blood cells, 12-22% contained in the plasma and approximately 3% contained in the leukocyte[202]. In 1990, Faur *et al*[203] reported that about 83% of serum zinc is loosely bound to albumin and 2% was gamma globulin bound while the rest serum zinc was bound strongly to $\alpha_2$-macroglobulin and transferrin to extent that they are not affected by sever alterations in serum zinc concentrations.

The most outstanding feature of the function of zinc is that it has a general stabilization effect on macromolecules, the II b transition metal, distinct from other essential trace metals in that it has only one valance state. It prevents the transfer of electrons from (oxidizing Compounds) free radicals to organic molecules in which it is found[204]. Zinc may exert its antioxidant effect by decreasing the susceptibility of essential sulfhydryl group of proteins to oxidation by competing with prooxidant metal such as iron and copper for biological binding sites[205]. Zinc is also an integral part of Cu-Zn- superoxide dismutase (Cu Zn SOD), a cytosolic or extracellular enzyme involved in the first line of defense against free radicals[206]. It was hypothesized that zinc deficiency impairs free radical defense and therefore cause tissue to be more susceptible to oxidation following exposure to oxidative stress[207], which result in damage to cellular structure and has been lined to many diseases including cancer[206].

Micro nutrients are able to influence the process of carcinogenesis by chemoprotective effects or the possible anticarcinogenic effects in the early stage of tumor development[208]. It is however an essential fact that the possible interaction between micro nutrients and carcinogenesis are complex problem that can not be considered by simple cause-effect relationship[208] the secretory epithelial cells of prostate gland have a unique function and capability of accumulating extremely high intracellular levels of zinc. One of the effects of this accumulation is inhibition of cell growth. The accumulation of high intracellular levels of zinc by prostate cells induces mitochondrial apoptogenesis. This may represent a physiological effect of zinc in the regulation of prostate cell growth[209].

It was found that the apoptosis-inducing activity of the purified apoptosis inducing protein was totally dependent on zinc. The depletion of zinc or substitution of zinc ion by barium was completely abolished the apoptosis-inducing activity of this protein which was found to inhibit prostate cancer in mice[210].

Zinc finger proteins are known to mediate various transcriptional control mechanisms and other cellular functions in human cells[211].

The amino peptidase-N (AP-N) enzymatic activity in relation to tumor cell invasion in human prostate had been proven. There is a strong suggestion that suppression of prostate cancer cell invasion by zinc was based on the inhibition of AP-N activity by zinc[212]. The effect of zinc on the invasion activity of human prostate and renal cancer cell were investigated in vitro using cell culture the invasive activity was effectively suppressed by zinc in a dose dependent manner[213].

# 2. Materials and Methods:

## 2.1 Chemicals:

1-$HNO_3$ (Fluka) analar grade.

2-$HCLO_4$ (Fluka) analar grade.

3-Standard solution of zinc saved in plastic container produced by Riedel-De Haen AG-Faxanal company.

## 2.2 Apparatus:

Atomic absorption spectrophotometer of type Perken-Elmer. 2380.

## 2.3 Patients:

The sera and tissue was obtained from the same patients whose mentioned in chapter two.

## 2.4 Samples collections and tissues preparation:

five milliliter of blood was with drawn from 31 patients with prostate cancer and 31 patients with BPH and 35 healthy individuals. The samples were centrifuged for 15 minute and the sera were obtained from each sample. The sera were frozen at $-20^0C$ till the time for use, before measurements the sera were kept at room temperature for several minutes to thaw. (The hemolysis samples were excluded from the group). Each 0.5 ml of serum was diluted ten times with a solution of

0.1% of KCl in deionized water. A portion of 20µl of the diluted serum was transferred by a suitable micropipette and injected into furnace tube for zinc determinations.

About 0.5g of each tissue samples was immersed in 25ml of a solution containing 10volumes of $HNO_3/HCLO_4(1:1)$[214]. After 72h in this solution the tissue was completely dissolved. The clear yellow solution was obtained and diluted ten times with deionized water. A 20µl of the diluted tissue solution was injected in the pore of the furnace tube of AAS for zinc determination.

## 2.5 Atomic Absorption Spectrophotometric Conditions for Zinc Measurements.

1-Electrodless discharge lamp of zinc was selected, connected and provided with suitable current 20mA for about 15 minute before starting the measurement to produce a stable resonance line.

2-The pore of the graphite furnace tube was turned and adjusted to be in a suitable position for injecting the samples.

3-All specific parameters of zinc which are illustrated in table (4-1) like wave length, band pass,.. etc was programmed[215]

4-Deuterium lump was used for back ground correction.

*Table (4-1): Instrumental Parameters of Flameless Atomic Absorption Spectrophotometer for Zinc.*[215]

| Parameter | Zn |
|---|---|
| Wave length (nm) | 213.9 |
| Spectral band pass (nm) | 0.7 |
| Lamp current (mA) | 20 |
| Volume of sample (ml) | 20 |
| Sheathing gas | Ar |
| Drying temp. ($C^0$) | 130 |
| Ashing temp. ($C^0$) | 400 |
| Atomization temp. ($C^0$) | 2300 |
| Drying time (s) | 40 |
| Ashing time (s) | 20 |
| Atomization time (s) | 3 |

## 2.6. Determination of Optimum Ashing Temperature.

1- Atomic absorption spectrophotometer was operated as illustrated in section 2.5.

2- The initial ashing temperature was selected to be $200C^0$. Then the temperature was gradually elevated and the absorbance was recorded at each temperature.

3- The absorbance which was decreased with temperature raise was recorded simultaneously.

4- The absorbance value were plotted against temperatures as illustrated in figure (4-1).

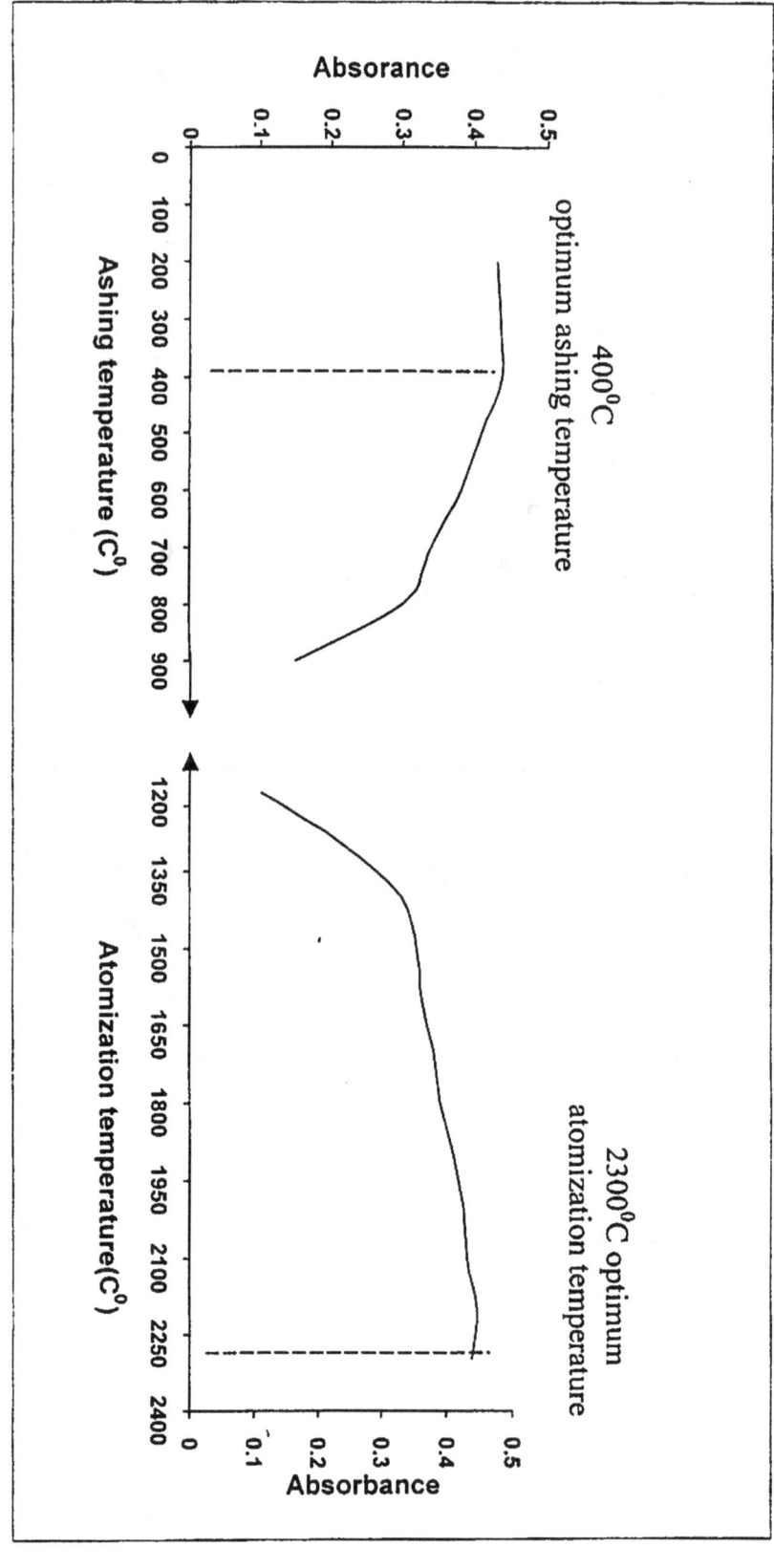

Figure (4-1): The optimum ashing and atomization temperature of zinc by flameless atomic absorption spectrophotometer. All other details are explained in the text.

## 2.7. Determination of Optimum Atomization temperature

1- Atomic Absorption spectrophotometer was operated as illustrated in section 2.5.

2- The initial atomization temperature was selected to be $1200C^0$ then the temperature was gradually elevated and the absorbance was recorded at each temperature

3- Absorbance values were plotted versus the temperature degrees as illustrated in figure (4.1).

## 2.8. Measurement of Zinc by Atomic Absorption Spectrophotometer

1- The standard solution of zinc was prepared with concentrations of 25, 50, 75, 100, 125, 150 $\mu g.l^{-1}$ from a stock solution of Riedel- De Hean Company.

2- Atomic absorption spectrophotometer was operated with zinc parameters as illustrated in section 2.5.

3- Twenty microliter of each sample or standard was injected through the port of the graphite furnace tube.

4- The sample was automatically dried, ashed and atomized when the measuring process operated.

5- Steps 2 and 3 were repeated three times with each sample.

6- The standard curve was obtained by plotting the absorbance values of standards against its concentrations as illustrated in figure (4-2).

7- The sensitivity of the method was $1.07 \times 10^{-8}$ M of zinc and the recovery was 98.84%

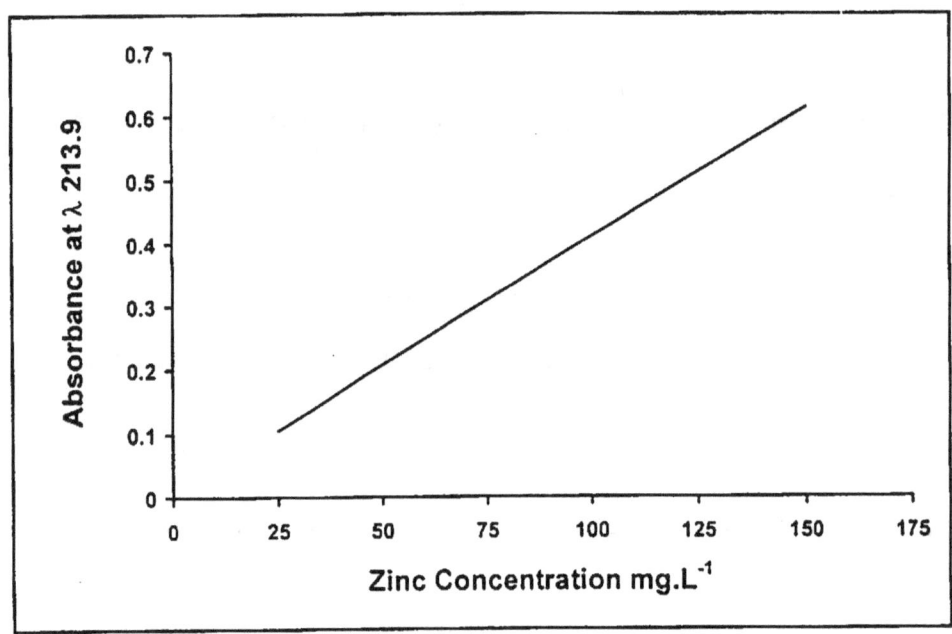

*Figure (4-2): Working standard curve for zinc determination by atomic absorption spectrophotometer. All other details are explained in the text.*

# 3. Result and Discussion

In clinical field, the use of atomic absorption spectrophotometer (AAS) as an analytical tool, has introduced precision and reliability in the determination of metals in biological fluids and tissues[216]. The electrothermal atomic absorption spectrophotometer was used in determination of zinc levels in sera and tissues of patients with prostate cancer and benign prostatic hyperplasia.

## 3.1. Serum Zinc level in Prostate cancer

Table (4-2) shows the mean values of sera zinc levels with the related statistical parameters.

*Table (4-2): Sera Zinc Levels in Prostate Cancer and Benign Prostatic Hyperplasia*

| Case | | Individual No. | Age range year | Serum Zinc μM | | |
|---|---|---|---|---|---|---|
| | | | | X | SD | CV% |
| Prostate cancer | Stage B | 11 | 55-75 | 11.2 | 2.4 | 21.4 |
| | Stage C | 13 | 57-72 | 10.5 | 2.82 | 26.9 |
| | Stage D | 7 | 60-75 | 10.4 | 2.98 | 28.7 |
| BPH | | 31 | 45-75 | 12.4 | 2.4 | 19.3 |
| control | | 35 | 45-75 | 11.85 | 1.92 | 16.2 |

The levels of zinc in sera of benign prostatic hyperplasia patients were significantly higher than that of controls. This enhancement may be concomitant with the second period of growth in prostate after 55years of old. The size of prostate gland increases during the first 20years of life, stabilize for further period about 35 year and then generally undergone a second period of growth[217]. Thus our result was in accordance with the speculation of Shamberger[218] who had mentioned that the enhancement of zinc level in patients with BPH may be considered as a useful index of the disease, especially when we refer to the role of zinc in the activity of those enzymes dealing with DNA, RNA and protein synthesis such as DNA polymerase, RNA polymerase and thymidine kinase.

In contrast, there is in general a significant decrease in mean values of serum zinc levels in prostate cancer in comparison with the mean value of healthy controls as shown in table (4-2).

The decrement of zinc level has been linked to many diseases including diabetes[219], abnormal immune function[222], cardiovascular diseases[221],and chronic liver disease[222]but Fenste et al[223] reported that serum zinc levels decrease in prostate cancer.

In table (4-2) the result of serum zinc level in three stages of prostate cancer was reported. Zinc in stage B was significantly higher than that of stage C and D and zinc level in stage D was significantly lower than stage C. This general decline in serum zinc level with cancer stage may be attributed to high demand on zinc for growth and proliferation of cancer cells. Zinc is necessary for DNA synthesis[224,225] since, its play a significant role in activation of the deoxythymidine kinase. Zinc also influence hormonal regulation of cell division[226]. The important role of zinc in growth suggested that it may be taken up by prostate cancer tissue and that result in zinc decrement in circulation.

## 3.2. Tissue Zinc level in Prostate Cancer

Zinc content of prostate tissue was measured by electrothermal atomic absorption spectrophotometeric method. Table (4-3) shows the concentration of tissue zinc in benign prostatic hyperplasia and prostate cancer. The results were compared with zinc levels in normal tissue that was obtained from the same patient of prostate cancer and was examined by the Pathologist for accurate histological diagnosis.

*Table (4-3): Tissue Zinc levels in Prostate Cancer and Benign Prostatic Hyperplasia*

| Tissue | | individual No. | Tissue Zinc level mg.g$^{-1}$ | | |
|--------|--|----------------|-------------------------------|--|--|
| | | | $\overline{X}$ | SD | CV% |
| Normal | | 16 | 108 | 10.3 | 9.5 |
| BPH | | 19 | 116 | 12.9 | 11.1 |
| Prostate Cancer | Stage B | 7 | 102 | 15.5 | 15.2 |
| | Stage C | 8 | 96 | 17.3 | 18.0 |
| | Stage D | 7 | 90 | 14.6 | 16.2 |

Table (4-3) shows that there is a significant enhancement in tissue zinc level of BPH in comparison with the levels of zinc in normal tissues. The high content of zinc may play a role in predisposition to BPH[227].

Zalewski *et al*[228] reported that there is a potential importance of zinc as an intercellular regulatory ion. Zinc involved in the regulation of cellular growth and differentiation including gene expression and in the regulation of apoptosis. Its thought that the transition metal Zn II regulate cell and tissue growth by enhancing mitosis (cell proliferation) and suppressing the counter balancing process of apoptosis (gene directed cell death)[229]. The accumulation of zinc in prostate gland may suggests that the zinc could be considered as a causative factor in BPH.

However Castello *et al*[230] investigation refers to the accumulation of zinc in prostate gland in case of BPH.

In contrast, table (4-3) shows a significant decrement in tissue zinc level in prostate cancer if compared with zinc level of normal tissue.

Tipton *et al*[231] reported that the normal value of zinc level in prostate gland was 102 $\mu g.g^{-1}$ of wet weight. Our result of zinc level in prostate cancer tissue was consistent with the result of Liang *et al*[232] They reported that zinc level in prostate cancer markedly lower than the level detected in non cancerous prostatic tissue. The results suggeste that the inhibition of human prostatic carcinoma cell growth, possibly due to induction of cell cycle arrest. The loss of unique capability to retain high levels of zinc in prostate gland is an important factor in the development of malignant prostate cells[232].

As shown in table (4-3) there is a differences in zinc levels with variation of the stages of prostate cancer. The decrement of zinc level with the raise in cancer stage may depend on the speculation of Castello *et al*[230]. The intramitochondrial accumulation of high zinc levels inhibits mitochondrial aconitase activity, which inhibits citrate oxidation. The inability of malignant prostate cells to accumulate high zinc levels results in increased citrate oxidation and ATP production which is essential for the progression of malignancy. Accordingly the decrement of zinc levels in prostate tissue was positively correlated with enhancement in prostate cancer stage to maintain the requirement of energy that needed for proliferation and growth during malignancy.

# General Discussion:

The IRMA method for total PSA determination was developed to produce a reaction that is characterized by the ability to reach an equilibrium point at certain time. The use of serum or tissue PSA and $^{125}$I-anti total PSA anti body was the development of choice in producing a reaction that convenient to follow the kinetics and thermodynamics of the PSA and to explore in vitro behavior of PSA toward its antibody.

Depending on the developed method and because the tissue of prostate cancer contained only the free PSA and no other immunologically active forms[193], it was easy to determine the kinetic and thermodynamic parameters of the binding of free PSA of prostate cancer tissue with $^{125}$I-anti total PSA anti body as mentioned in chapter two, but Prakash *et al*[233] reported that a notable difference in immunoreactivity between free PSA isolated from seminal fluid and free PSA which isolated from serum. Moreover, Blasé *et al*[234] reported that there is a different affinity and reaction kinetics with free PSA isolated from serum and that from seminal fluid, hence the attention was paid to make a comparison between serum free-PSA and the free PSA of prostate cancer tissue in kinetics and thermodynamics fields.

The free PSA in the circulation does not existed alone, but it is combined with other immunologically active forms of PSA. The PSA which associated with the protein $\alpha_1$-antichymotrypsin (ACT) is the most abundant isoform of PSA in the circulation, while the free PSA is the minor component[25]. Both of them have the ability to react with the available antibody, but which of them have the ability to react faster than the other toward the desired antibody?.

To over take this point, it was necessary to separate the free PSA from the combined PSA with ACT in order to maintain a reliable manner to make an accurate comparison between the free PSA of the tissue of prostate cancer and free PSA of the serum of prostate cancer and get rid of all the interference that may caused by the presence of PSA-ACT in the reaction media. The separation was achieved successfully using the gel Sephadex G-150 due to the high differences in the molecular weight between the two species and then the isolated free PSA from sera of patients with prostate cancer was obtained alone.

The kinetic and thermodynamic parameters were determined for the reaction between free PSA isolated from sera and the $^{125}$I-anti total PSA anti body and then compared with those obtained from tissue PSA. The comparability of the kinetics and thermodynamics results of the two species reflects the close similarity in structure between them.

Now, depending on these results and with consideration for Prakash *et al*[233] speculations, it is possible to conclude that there is a notable difference in immunoreactivity between free PSA isolated from the semen and free PSA in the cancerous prostatic tissue.

The value of free PSA to total PSA ratio was calculated in different stages of prostate cancer. Although the free PSA to total PSA ratio differentiated well between benign and malignant diseases[89], there is a lack of correlation between the calculated free PSA to total PSA ratios and cancer stages.

The search for a reasons that may account for the fluctuations of serum free PSA to total PSA ratios in different stages of prostate cancer led to investigation the role of the zinc.

It was reported that zinc could play a role in preventing the formation of PSA-ACT complex, likewise the disappearance of this complex in prostatic fluids and seminal plasma was attributed to the high concentration of zinc in these sites[30], so that the zinc was investigated to estimate its role in the alteration of the free PSA to total PSA ratio instead of the previous factor which was the stage of prostatic cancer.

Zinc analysis which was performed by the electrothermal atomic absorption spectrophotometric method manifested the high significant differences in zinc level between sera and tissues of prostate cancer. On the other hand the lack of correlation ($r = -0.97$) between serum zinc level in different stages of prostate cancer and the values of the free PSA to total PSA ratio that mentioned in table (5-1) revealed that there is other factors might be responsible for the alterations of free PSA to total PSA ratio.

*Table (5-1): Sera Zinc Levels and Free PSA to Total PSA Ratios of Patients with Different Stages of Prostate Cancer.*

| Prostate Cancer Stage | Serum Zinc (μM) | f-PSA / t-PSA % |
|---|---|---|
| B | $11.2 \pm 2.40$ | 11.34 |
| C | $10.5 \pm 2.82$ | 13.78 |
| D | $10.4 \pm 2.98$ | 13.50 |

The two factors that were investigated during this work the cancer stages and serum zinc levels, unfortunately were'nt well correlated with the values of free PSA to total PSA ratios which were obtained from sera of patients with prostate cancer. Further works, may be necessary to understand the biological interactions between PSA and ACT and the factors that may influence the free PSA total PSA ratio in sera of patients with prostate cancer. The other important point is that the PSA was considered for a long time as a factor that aid to precipitate cancer. In 1995 James *et al*[235] emphasized on a putative fact that human PSA is a secreted antigen and should be taken into consideration, its potential use as a target for human prostate cancer and as a secreted antigen may also reduce immunoglobulin responses by forming antigen-antibody complexes and/or potentially restraining specific T-cells responses. In the same direction Etsuo *et al*[143] reported that in prostate cancer PSA may play an important role in the invasion and metastatic processes as an initiator of malignancy.

In contrast to these speculations our results show that the levels of PSA in non cancerous tissues were higher than PSA levels in cancerous prostatic tissue with a percent of 31%.

Our results were corroborated by Eleftherios *et al*[145] speculations. They mentioned that the PSA should be considered as a cancer fighter at the tissue level and a valuable messenger (indicator) at the level of systematic circulation.

## Conclusions:

* The development protocol for the assay of PSA is suitable for the assessment of PSA in tissue.

* Serum PSA levels in Iraqi population seem to be higher than those reported in USA and western European countries and that may be attributed to the early detection of prostate cancer due to the widely use of PSA as a screening test in these countries.

* The use of PSAD doesn't improve the PSA ability in predicting prostate cancer in the used levels of PSA in this study.

* The effort to produce cancers vaccines or therapies targeting PSA expression is the wrong strategy and the PSA should be considered as a cancer fighter and the effort should be directed toward over expression of PSA at tissue level.

* Kinetics studies on PSA of prostate cancer tissue binding with $^{125}$I-anti total PSA antibody revealed that the binding reaction is temperature and time dependent while binding data fits the pseudo first order reaction kinetics.

* Thermodynamic parameters of the binding of PSA of prostate cancer tissue with $^{125}$I-anti total PSA antibody reveals that the non-covalent reaction was entropically driven and $\Delta H^0$ contribution to the stability of the product was very low.

* The free PSA/ total PSA ratios are no additional value in prediction of prostate cancer stage.

* Serum free PSA of prostate cancer is very close in structure to the tissue PSA of prostate cancer, the fact that was concluded from the comparability of kinetic and thermodynamic parameters of both species.

* The complex PSA-ACT is not existed in prostatic tissue , while it is the predominant form of PSA in circulation. This fact may attribute to the high level of zinc in prostate tissue.

* The clinical importance of PSA level in evaluating outcome was reduced to large extent at first three weeks after surgery.

# The future works:

According to the results obtained throughout this thesis, the following works are suggested for the future:

* Determination of PSAD at ranges of PSA lower to those reported in this thesis and exploration of its addition to the ability of PSA to discriminate between prostate cancer and BPH.

* Determination of the kinetic and thermodynamic parameters of the seminal PSA and compare them with those obtained from sera and tissues to assess the comparability in structure of PSA isoforms in these sites during prostate cancers.

* Determination of free PSA to total PSA ratios in other diseases of prostate gland or other types of prostate cancer.

* Exploration of the ability of zinc to dissociate the complex between PSA and ACT.

# References

1- Belonger A, Rang PM, Liu S: Clin. Invest. Med. 1993; **16(6)**: 409-412.

2- Ambruster D. A: Clin. Chem. 1993; **39**: 181-185.

3- Wang M, Papsiderol, Kuriyama M: Prostate. 1981; **2**: 89-96.

4- Lilja H. World: J. Urol. 1993; **11**: 188-91.

5- Robert M., Gibbs BF: Biochemistry 1997; **36**: 3811-9.

6- Lundwall A, Lilja H: FEBS Lett 1987; **214**: 317-22.

7- Hara M, Koyanagi Y, Inoue T: Jpn. J. Legal med. 1971; **25**: 322-5.

8- Li T, Beling C: Fertil Steril. 1973; **24**: 134-6.

9- Wang M, ValenzuelaL, Murphy G: Invest. Urol. 1979; **17**: 159.

10- Papsidero L, Wang M, Valenzuela L: Cancer Res. 1980; **40**: 2428.

11- Chan DW, Sokoll LJ: JIFCC. 1997; **9**: 120-5.

12- Neal DJ, Clejan S, Sarma D:.Prostate 1992; **148**: 83-7.

13- Hudson MA, Bahnson RR, Catalona WJ: J. Urol. 1989; 7: 7-11.

14- Benson MC, Whang IS, Pantuk A: J. Urol. 1992; **147**: 815-9.

15- Carter HB, Morrel CH, Pearson JD: Cancer Res. 1992; **52**: 3323-7.

16- Oesterling JE, Jacobsen SJ, Chute CG: J. Am. Med. Assoc. 1993; **270**: 860-3.

17- Stenman UH, Leinoner J, Alfthan H: Cancer Res. 1991; **51**: 222-7.

18- Gerhard M., Ulrich B: Clin. Chem. 1996; **42**: 691-5.

19-Brower M. K., Rennels M. A: Amer. J. Clin Path. 1988; **89**: 428-32.

20-Graves HC, *et al*: Clin. Chem. 1995; **41**: 7-9.

21-Webber MM, Waphray A, Bello D: Clin. Cancer Res. 1995; 1: 089-1094.

22-Sutkowiski DM, Goode Rl, Baniel J, Teater C, Cohem P, Mc Nulty AM: J. Natl. cancer Inst. 1999; **91**: 1663-1669.

23-Stein A, Dekernion JB, Smith RB: J. Urol. 1992; **147**: 942-7.

24-Diamandis EP, Yu H: J. Clin. Endocrinol. Metab. 1995; **80**: 1515-1517.

25-Lilja H, Christensson A, Pahlein V: Clin. Chem. 1991; **37**: 1618.

26-Zhang WM, Finne P, Leinonen J, Vesalainen S, Nordling S, Rannikko S, Stenman VH: Clin Chem. 1998; **44**: 2471-9.

27-Blanger A, Rong PM, Lin S: Clin. Inves. Med. 1993; **16**: 409-44.

28-Christensson A, Bjok T, Nilsson O: J. Urol. 1993; **150**: 100-3.

29-Stenman UH, Leinonem J, Alfthan H, Rannikkos, Tuhkanen, Cancer Res. 1991; **51**: 22-6

30-Yi Q, Julia AS, David JZ, Harry GR:. Clin. Chem. 1997; **43**: 352-9.

31-Oesterling JE, Jacobsen SJ, Klee GG: J. Urol. 1995; **154**: 1090-4.

32-Luderer AA, Chen YT, Soriano TF: Urology. 1995; **46**: 187-93.

33-Brande D., Kircheim D, Scott W. Ultrastructure of the human Prostate: Normal and Neoplastic. Lab Inves 1996.

34-Stamey MD, Mc Neal JE. Adenocarcinoma of prostate. In: Walsh P, RetikA, StameyT etal. Campbell's urology ed6. Philadelphia: WB saunders 1992:**1185**.

35-Isaacs Jt, Lundmo pl, Bergers R: Prostate, 1983; **4**:351-7.

36-Bonkhoff H, Remberger K: Prostate. 1996; **28**: 98-102.

37-Ramela J. R, suzannme B., Phillip S: Clinical Chemistry, 1998; **44**: 705-723.

38-Gunther HJ, Rundolf H, Prostate cancer, Williams and Wilkins Baltimore, London 1980.

39-Ballentine Carter H, piantadosi S, Isaacs JT: J. Urol. 1990; **143**: 742.

40-Kirby RS, Christmas TJ, Brawer M. In: Prostate cancer. M. Mosbey. London, 1996.

41-Catalona W. J: N. Engl. J. Med. 1994; **331**: 996-1004.

42-Keetch DW, Humphery PA, Smith DS, Stahl D, Catalona WJ: J. Urology. 1996; **155**: 1841-3.

43-Smith DS, Bullock AD, Catalona WJ, Herschman JD: J. Urology. 1996; **156**: 1366-9.

44-Morton MS, Geriffith K, Black Look N: Br. J. Urol. 1996; **77**: 481-93.

45-Vander Gulden JM, Verbeek AL, Kolk JJ: Br. J. Urol, 1994; **73**: 382-9.

46-Hanchette C. L., Schwart z G. G: Cancer 1992; **70**: 2861-9.

47-Borre M, Nerstmom B, Overgaad J: Cancer. 1997; **80**; 917-28.

48-Gihes R.F *et al*: N.Engl. J. Med. 1991; **324**: 236-45.

49-Greenlee RT, Murray T, Boldem S, Wingo PA: CA cancer J. Clin. 2000; **50**: 7-33.

50-Results of Iraqi cancer registry-Iraq cancer Board-Ministry of health.

51-Stamey TA, Mc Neal JE, adenocarcinoma of the prostate in: Walsh P, Retik A, stamey T etal, Compbell's Urology ed6. Philadelphia: W.B. Saunders, **1992**: 1159.

52-Ro JY, Tetu B, Ayala AG: Cancer 1987; **59**: 977-81.

53-Ginesin Y, Bokein M, Moskovitz B: Eur. Urol. 1986; **12**: 441-5.

54-Murphy G P, Gaeta J F, pickren J., Wajsman Z: Cancer 1980; **45**: 1889.

55-Levran Z., Ganzlez JA, Diokno AC:.Br. J Urol. 1995; **75**: 778-82.

56-Rifkin MD, Zerhouni EA, Gatsonis CA: N. Engl. J. Med. 1990; **323**: 621-35.

57-Gleason DF: Hum. Pathol. 1992; **75**: 574.

58-Stamey TA: Urology 1995; **45**: 563-8.

59-Stamey TA, Freiha FS, Mc Neal JE: Cancer; 1993; **71**: 933-37.

60-Pollack HM, Schnall MD: Prostate 1992; **4**: 19-23.

61-Litwin MS, Hays RD, Fink A: JAMA. 1995; **273**: 129-35.

62-Irving D. K., Richard Sc., Malcolm AB: J. Ural. 1993; **149**: 519-22.

63-Sokeland J.; Urology A Poket Reference; 2nd .ed: Thieme Flexi Book; 1989; PP: 254.

64-Cox RL, Crawford ED: J. Urol 1995; **154**: 1991-7.

65-Devoogt HJ, Smith PH: J. Urol. 1986; **135**: 303.

66-MC Connell JD: Urol Clin North. Am. 1991; **18**: 1-4.

67-Havlin KA, Trump DL: Cancer Treat Res 1988; **39**: 83-7.

68-Schell hammer P, Sharifi R, Block N: Urology 1995; **45**: 745-9.

69-Denis LJ, Carneiro de Moura JL, Bono A:Urology, 1993; **42**: 119-23.

70-Klapdor R. Malignant tumors of the liver in: Tumor markers in clinical oncology an over view 2nd ed. Sorin biomedica 1993. pp3.

71-Joseph O, Zvi F, Cheryl L, Howard S. cancer of the prostate in: Cancer principle and practice of oncology part2. 5th ed 1997. pp. 1339.

72-Gutman EB, Sproul EE, Gutman AB: AM. J. Cancer 1996; **28**: 485-9.

73-Burtis CA, Ashwood ER; Teitze Text Book of Clinical Chemistry 2nd ed; W. B. Sounder company 1994.

74-Tewari P. C. Williams JS: Clin.. Chem. 1998; **44**: 191-7.

75-Peehl DM: Prostate. 1996; **6**: 74-78.

76-Takayam TK, Fujikawa K: J. Biol. Chem.1997; **272**: 21582-8.

77-Pirkko V: Eur. Urol. 1995; **27** (suppl2):4.

78-Sandrine M, Gilbert D, Jean PC, Jacques P: Clin. Chem. 1999; **45**: 638-650.

79-Nixon RG, Brawer MK: Urol. 1996; **9**: 1-8.

80-Osterling JE *et al*: J. Urol. 1988; **139**: 766-71.

81-Peehl DM, *et al*: Cancer 1995; **75**: 2021-6.

82-Benson MC: J. Urol. 1994; **152**: 2046-8.

83-Fichtner J, Graves HC, thatcherK, YemotoC: J. Urol. 1996; **155**: 738-742.

84-Pauliina N., Ville V., Timo P., Lilija H: Clin Chem. 2000; **46**: 1610-1618.

85-Stemman UH, Leinonen J, Altthan H, Rannikko S, Tuhkanen K, Alfthan: Cancer Res. 1991; **51**: 222-6.

86-David GB: Eur. Urol. 1995; **27**: 5-9.

87-Kimberly L. B., David G. B: J. Ural. 1994; **151**: 1565-70.

88-Irving D, Richard S, Malcolm A: J. Urol. 1993; **149**: 519-22.

89-Pearson JD, Luderer AA, Metter EJ: Urology 1996; **48**: 4-8.

90-Bjok T, Bjartell A, lilja H: Urol. 1994; **43**: 427-34.

91-Lianidou ES, Angelopoulou K, Katsarros D, Durando A, Massobrio M: Clin Biochem. 1998; **31**: 551-553.

92-Mettlin Cm, Littrup PJ, Kane RA: Cancer 1991; **74**: 1615.

93-Brwaer MK, Chetner MP, Beatie J: J. Urol. 1992; **147**: 841-45.

94-Crawford ED, de Antoni EP: Urol. Clin. N. Am. 1993; **20**: 637-40.

95-Cooner W. H: Urol. Clin. N. Am. 1993; **20**: 575-9.

96-Brawer MK: CA. Cancer. J. Clin. 1995; **45**: 148-51.

97-Littrap PJ., Kane RA, Mettlin CJ: Cancer 1994; **74**: 3146-49.

98-Hanley JA, Mc Neil BJ: Radiology 1982; **143**: 29-35.

99-Kimberly L. B, David G. B., Robert PM:.J. Urol. 1994; **151**: 565-70.

100-Benson M C, Whang IS, Olsson CA: J. Urol. 1992; **147**: 817-21.

101-Seamon E, Whang M, Olsson CA: Urol. Clin. N. Am. 1993; **20**: 653-8.

102-Carter H. B, Pearson JD: Urol. Clin. N. Amer. 1993; **20**: 665-8.

103-Carter H. B, Pearson J, Wacliwew X: J. Urol. 1994; **151**: 312-17.

104-Carter H. B, Pearson J, Metter JE: J. AM. Med Assoc. 1992; **267**: 2215-9.

105-Dalkin BL, Ahmann F, Sowthwick P, Bottaccini MR: J. Urol. 1993; **149**: 413.

106-Oesterling JE, Cooner WH, Jacobsen SJ: Urol. Clin. N. AM. 1993; **20**: 371-6.

107-Richie JP, Catalona WJ, Ahman FR: J. Urol. 1993; **42**: 365-8.

108-Oesterling JE, Cooner WH, Jacobsen SJ: Urol. Clin. N. AM. 1993; **20**: 671-4.

109-Petteway J, Brawer MK: J. Urol. 1995; **153**: 465.

110-El-Galley RE, Petros JA, Sanders WH: Urology 1995; **46**: 200.

111-Nixon R G, Brawer MK: Urology 1996; **9**: 18-23.

112-Cooner WH, Mosley BR, Rutherford Cl: J. Urol. 1990; **143**: 1146-50.

113-Littrup P, Goodman A, Mettlin C: Cancer 1992; **42**: 198-201.

114-Babaian RJ, Dinney CR, Ramirez EL: Urology 1993; **41**: 421-7.

115-Mc Cormack RT, Ritteuhouse HG, Finlay JA. Urology 1995; **45**: 729-35

116-Stamey TA, Kabalin JN: J. Urol. 1989; **141**: 1070.

117-Partin A, Yoo J, Carter HB: J. Urol. 1993; **150**: 110-14.

118-Dupont A, CusanL, Gomez JL, Thibeault M. M, Tremblay M: J. Urol. 1991; **146**: 1064-1068.

119-Lindstedt G., Jacobsson A: Clin. Chem. 1990; **361**: 53-58.

120-Stein A, Dekeanion JB: J. Urol. 1992; **147**: 942-6.

121-Oesterling JE: J. Urol. 1991; **145**: 907- 923.

122-Lilja H,Christensson A,Dahlen V, Matikanem MY, Nilon O, Pettersson K: Clin. Chem. 1991; **37**: 1618-25.

123-Becker C., lilja H. Clin. Chem. Acta. 1997; **257**: 117-32.

124-Patfox M, Andrew AR, Erasmus S: Clin. Chem. 1999; **45**: 1181-1189.

125-Burtis C A, Ashwood ER, Teitze Text Book of Clinical Chemistry; 2nd ed: W. B Sounders Company: 1994.

126-Chan DW, Bruzek DJ, Oesterling JE, Rock RC, Walsh PC: Clin. Chem.1987; **33**: 1916-20.

127-Kleer E, Dodge LA, Zincke H: J. Urol. 1994; **115**: 94-8.

128-Lowry DH, Rose brough NJ, Farr Al: J. Biol. Chem. 1951; **93**: 265-8.

129-Emil A.T, Jack W.W., Smith's General Urology. 14ed. Appleton and Lange. Calisornia. 1992. PP: 388.

130-Elgalley RE, Peteros JA, Sanders WH: Urology 1995; **46**:200.

131-Petteway J, Brower M. K: J. Urol. 1995; **153**: 465.

132-Irani J, Millet C., Levillain P: Eur. Urol. 1998; **29**: 407-412.

133-Oesterling JE, Partin AW, Polascik TJ: J. Urol. 1999, **162**: 293-3-6.

134-Cupp MR, Oesteraling JE: Mayo. Clin. Proc. 1993; **68**: 297-303.

135-Benson Mc, Whang IS, Olsson CA: J. Urol. 1992; **147**: 817-22.

136-Stamey TA, Yang N, Hay AR, Mc Neal JE: N. Engl. J. Med. 1987; **317**: 909-16.

137-Frazier A, Robertson JE, Humphrey PA: J. Urol. 1993; **149**: 150-6.

138-Oesterling JE, Chan DW, Epstein JI: J. Urol; 1991; **139**: 907-12.

139-Lindstedt G, Jacobson A, Lundberg A, Hedelin H: Clin. Chem. 1990; **36**: 53-58.

140-Stein A, Dekernion JB, Dorey F: Brit. J. Urol. 1991; **67**: 626-31.

141-Partin AW, Pound CR, Clemenus TQ, Epstein JI, Walsh PC: Urol. Clin. N. Amer. 1993; **20**: 713-16.

142-Pirkko Vihko: Eur. Urol. 1995; **27** (suppl2): 4.

143-Etsuo Y, Sayuri O, Masahiko S, Masugi M, Hisashi M: Int. J. Cancer 1995; **63**: 383-5.

144-Dawid G. Bost Wick: E. Urol. 1995; **27**: 5-8.

145-Eleftherios P. Diamand IS: Clinical Chemistry 2000; **46**: 896-900.

146-Fortier AH, Nelson BJ, Grella DK, Holaday JW: Br. J. Cancer. 1999; **81**: 1269-1273.

147-Heidtmann HH, Nettel beck DM, Mingles A, Jager R, Weker HG: J. Natl. Cancer Inst. 1999; **19**: 1635-1640.

148-Ferdinardo M, Maurizio S, Silvana A: Clin. Chem. 1997; **43**: 1148-54.

149-Malm J, Helman J, Hogg P, Lilja H: Prostate 2000: **45**: 132-9.

150-Hsieh MC, Cooperman BS: Biochem. Biophys. Acta. 2000; **1481**: 75-87.

151-Laurant T. C: Biochem. J. 1963; **89**: 249.

152-Seeley DH, Wang WY, Salhanick HA: Biochem Biophys Acta. 1980; **632(4):** 536.

153-Wealbroeck M, Van-obberghen E, De-Meyter P: J. Biol. Chem. 1979; **254**: 7736.

154-Nemthy G, Scheraga HA: J. Phys. Chem. 1962; **66**: 1773.

155-Ross PD, Subramarian N: Biochemistry 1981; **20**: 3096-9.

156-Harol S, Talamantes FJ: Mol. Cell. Endocrinol. 1985; **43**: 199-203.

157-Christensson A, Biork T, Nilsson D: J. Urol. 1993; **150**: 100-5.

158-Bangma CH, Kranse R, Blijenberg PG, Schroder FH: J. Urol. 1997; **157**: 544-7.

159-Elgamal AA, Cornillie FJ, Van Poppel H. P, Van de Voorde MW. Mc Cabe R, Baert LV: J. Urol. 1996; **156**: 1042-7.

160-Toubert ME, Guillet J, Chiron M, Meria P, Role C., Schlogeter MH: Eur. J. Cancer 1996; **32**: 2088-93.

161-Van Cangh PJ, Denyer P, Saunage P, Tombal B: Prosetate 1996; **7**: 30-4.

162-Christensson A, Bjor K A, Nilsson O, Dahlen U: Urology, 1994; **43**: 427-34.

163-Espana F, Royo M, Martine ZM, Enguidaues MJ: J. Urol. 1998; **160**: 2081-8.

164-Lilja H, Christensson A, Dahlen V, Maitikaninen M. T, Nilson B. Pettersson K: Clin. Chem. 1991; **37**: 1618-25.

165-Wu JT, Wilson L, Zhang P, Meikle AW, Stephenson R: J. Clin. Anal. 1995; **9**: 15-24.

166-Allard WJ, Zhov Z, Yeung KK: Clin. Chem. 1998; **44**: 1216-23.

167-Michael N, Klaus J, Ulrike E, Tobias P, CarstenS, Brigitte B: Eur. Urol. 2001; **34**: 57-64.

168-Piironen T, Villoutreix BO, becker C, Holling Sowrth K: Protein. Sci. 1998; **7**: 259-69.

169-Frankle AE, Rouse RV, Wang MC, Chu TM: Cancer Res. 1982; **42**: 3714-8.

170-Petterssonk, Pilronen T, Sepala M, Liukkonen L: Clin. Chem, 1995; **41**: 1480-8.

171-Nilsson O, Peter A, Andersson I, Nilssonk, Groundstrom B: Br. J. Cancer 1997; **75**: 789-97.

172-Corey E, Wanger SK, Stray JE, Corey MJ: Int. J. Cancer 1997; **71**: 1019-28.

173-Jette DC, Kreutz FT, malcolm BA, Wishart DS: Clin. Chem. 1996; **42**: 1961-9.

174-Corey E, Wenger SK, Corey MJ, Vessella RL: Clin. Chem. 1997; **43**: 575-84.

175-Ferdinando M, Maurizio S, Silvana A, Giancarlo G: Clin. Chem. 1997; **43**: 1448-54.

176-Klaus J, Brigitte B, Michael L: Clin Chem. 2000; **46**: 47-54.

177-Scopes R, Protein Purification principles and practice. Springer Verlay New York. Heidelber Berlin. 1982. PP. 162.

178-Sanderine M, Gilbert D, Jean P, Nicole B: Clinical Chemistry 1999; **45**: 638-650.

179-Russel J. W, Quentin NM, Nancy N. P. Fundamentals of immunology for student of medicine and related sciences. Lea and Febiger-Philadelphia USA. 1982.

180-Lilja Hr Dahlen V: Clinical Chemistry. 1991; **37**: `618-22.

181-Wang MC, Papsidero LC, Kuriyama M: Prostate 1981; **12**:89-96.

182-Christensson A, Laurell CB, Lilija H: Eur. J. Biochem. 1990; **194**: 755-9.

183-Lilija H: Urol. Clin. North. Am. 1993; **20**: 681-5.

184-Wang Mc, valen Znela LA, Murply GP: Invest. Urol. 1979; **17**: 159-63.

185-Armbruster DA: Clin. Chem. 1993; **39**: 181-95.

186-Daniele M, Andrea B, Alberto R, Lisy G: Urologia Inter Nationalis. 2001; **67**: 272-282.

187-Lilja H, Curestensson A, Dahlen V: Clin. Chem. 1991; **37**: 1618-22.

188-Stenman UH, Leinonen J, Alfthan H: Cancer. Res. 1991; **51**: 222-6.

189-Charis HB, Reisk, Bert GB, Fritiz S: J. Urol. 1997; **157**: 544-547.

190-Jochen P, Carlo U, Wolfgang H: Clin. Chem. 2000; **46**: 474-482.

191-Allard WJ, Zhou Z, Yeung KK: Clin. Chem. 1998; **48**: 1216-23.

192-Van SM, Van CK: Urol. Res. 1983; **11**: 275-7.

193-Zhang WM, Finne P, Leinonen J, Vesalainen S: Clin. Chem. 1999; **45**: 814-21.

194-Michael P, Andrew W, Organic and Bio-Organic mechanisms. Addison Wesley longman. 1997, P6.

195-Mengle K, Kirkby EA. Zinc in nutrition in: Principle of plant nutrition pp. 533-535.

196-Underwood EJ. Zinc in: Trace element in human and animals nutrition. pp. 196-247.

197-Failla ML. Zinc function and transport in microorganism in: Microorganism and minerals. pp. 159-214. Marcel Dekker, New York. 1977.

198- Prasad AS, biochemistry of zinc. Plenum press. New York 199.

199- Coleman E: Ann v. Rev. Biochem 1992; **61**: 897-946.

200-Solomons N. W. zinc and copper in: Modern nutrition in health and disease. ME. Shils. Ed7. 1987.

201-Vallee B. L., Auld DS: Biochem. 1990; **29**:5647-59.

202-Robert C, Anonda S.P., Parviz IR, Zafallah T.C: Clin. Chem. 1982; **28**:475-80.

203-Faur H, Favier A, Tripier M, Arnand J: Biol. Trace. Elem. Res. 1990; **24**:25-37.

204-Hammer muller JD, Bary TM, Bettger W. J: J. Nutr. 1987; **117**: 894-8.

205- Bray T.M, Bettger WJ: Free Rad. Biol. Med. 1990; **8**:281-91.

206- Bostwick DG, Alexander EE, Stantella RM, Oberly LW: Cnccer. 2000; **89**:123-35 .

207-Leavy MA, Nose MD, Iles K, Bray TM, Trace element in man and animal. NRC Research press. Ottawa-Canada pp333-6.

208-Markt LW: Forsch-Komplement aremed. J. 1999; **6**:248-55.

209-Feng P, Liang JY, Fran klin R, Coslell K: Mol. Urol. 2000; **4**:31-6.

210-Tsai MH, Yu GL: Cancer 2001; **106**: 173-84.

211-Matak A, Murakami T, Wada Y, Tsu Tsumis: J. Atheroscler-thromb. 2000; 7:97-103.

212-Hirano K, sugimura Y, Hioki T, Usui S: Int. J. Cancer. 2001; **92**: 49-54.

213-Lshi k, Yamamato H, Sugimura Y: Biol. Pharm. Bull. 2001; **24**:226-30.

214-Ehnd J.M, Joseph GS, Mordechai C: Cancer 1983; **52**:868-72.

215-Perkin E. Clinical method for atomic absorption spectroscopy Perkin Elemer Company Connecticut 1973.

216-Lee K, Jacob E: Micro Chimica. Acta. 1974; **1**:65-75.

217-Mckenzie M.J: Amer. J. Clin. Nutr. 1979; **32**:570-9.

218-Shamberger RJ, Nutrition and cancer, clinical foundation. 2ed. Ohio, Pelenum press. New York and London (1984).

219-Cas N, Cas A, Granic M, Skrabalo Z, Moucilivic B: Biol. Trace element. Res. 1992; **32**:325-9.

220-Allen J.I Kay NE, Mc Clain C.J. Minne M: Annals of Internal. Medicine 1981; **95**:154-9.

221-Anderson RA: Acta. Pharmacol. Toxicol. Copenh. 1986; **59**: 317-24.

222-Capacaccia L, Merli M, Piat C, Servi R, Zullo A, Riggo O: Ital. J. Gastroenterol. 1991; **23**:386-9.

223-Fenste L, Wennirch R., Schmidt B: Urol. Res. 1989; **17**:14-17.

224-Chester JK, Petrie L, Tranis AJ: Biochem. J. 1990; **272**: 525-7.

225-Chester JK, Petrie L, Lipson KE: J. Cell. Physiology. 1993; **155**: 445-51.

226-Roth H. P, Kirchgessner M: J. Anim. Phys. Anim. Nutr. 1997; **77**:91-101.

227- Cousins R.J: Proc. Nutr. Soc. 1998; **57**:307-11.

228-Zalewski PD, Forbes IJ, Seamark RF, Borling hous R, Bett WH. Lincolin SF: Chem. Biol. 1994; **1**:153-61.

229-Ruth S. Mc Donald: J.Nutr. 2000; **130**:1500-8.

230-Castello LC, Franklin RB: Prostate. 1998; **35**: 285-96.

231-Tipton IH, Cook MJ: Health Phys. 1963; **9**:103-9.

232-Liang JY, Liu YY, Zan J, Franklin RB: Prostate. 1990; **40**:200-7.

233-Prakash CT, Julie SW, Clin. Chem. 1998; 44: 191-2.

234-Blasé AB, Sokoloff RL, Smith KM. Clin. Chem. 1997; 43: 843-5.

235-James WH, Jeffrey S, Susan JD Joseph ET, Clyde WW: Int. J. Cancer. 1995; 63: 231-37.

# CONTENTS

| Subject | Page no. |
|---|---|

| Subject | Page no. |
|---|---|

www.ingramcontent.com/pod-product-compliance
Lightning Source LLC
Chambersburg PA
CBHW081149180526
45170CB00006B/1995